The New National Health
Organization and Management

Chris Ham
Fellow in Health Policy and Management
King's Fund College

With a foreword by
Duncan Nichol

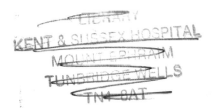

RADCLIFFE MEDICAL PRESS
OXFORD

British Library Cataloguing in Publication Data
Ham, Christopher
The new National health service: organization and management
1. Great Britain. National health service
I. Title
362.10941
ISBN 1 870905 96 2

Printed and bound in Great Britain
Typeset by Advance Typesetting Ltd, Oxfordshire

Contents

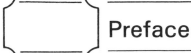

Preface

This book is intended to provide an introduction to the NHS. It contains basic information about the organization and financing of health services, management arrangements, and health care policies. Most of this information relates to England. Differences in the organization of health services in the rest of the United Kingdom are discussed in chapter 2. Suggestions for further reading are included for readers who would like additional information.

Thanks are due to the many individuals who commented on an earlier draft, and to the Department of Health for helping to support publication.

CHRIS HAM
King's Fund College
London
November 1990

Note on terminology

Throughout the handbook, Regional Health Authorities (RHAs), District Health Authorities (DHAs), and Special Health Authorities (SHAs) are referred to as health authorities. The term National Health Service (NHS) authorities is used to describe these authorities and family health services authorities (FHSAs). NHS Trusts (NHSTs) are not included in the description NHS authorities.

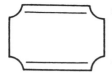# Foreword

The NHS is about to embark on the most challenging of reforms. They offer enormous potential for improving the quality of service to patients and for ensuring the NHS operates in as efficient and effective a way as possible.

A particular responsibility lies upon the members/directors of Family Health Services Authorities, health authorities and NHS Trusts. The leadership and direction they can give, ensuring that the NHS is working to clear objectives in delivering services to patients, is essential to the success of the reforms.

In order to carry out this role, members/directors need to be as well-informed as possible. I am delighted therefore to congratulate NAHAT and the King's Fund College on their initiative and hard work in producing this book. I am sure that all who read it will find it both useful and informative.

D K NICHOL
Chief Executive
NHS Management Executive

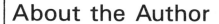

About the Author

Chris Ham is a Fellow at the King's Fund College. He has held posts at the universities of Bristol and Leeds and at the King's Fund Institute. His academic qualifications include a BA and M Phil from the University of Kent and a PhD from the University of Bristol. He is the author of five books including *Health Policy in Britain* and *Health Check: Health Care in an International Context*. Chris works closely with chairmen and members of health authorities and with senior managers. As well as his work in the UK, he has been involved in health services in Sweden, Finland, New Zealand, Spain, The Netherlands, West Germany, and France. Chris is married with three children and lives in north London.

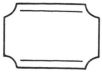 # National Association of Health Authorities and Trusts

The National Association of Health Authorities and Trusts (NAHAT) came into being on 1 August 1990, formed from a merger of the National Association of Health Authorities and the Society of Family Practitioner Committees.

NAHAT's primary role is to express the collective views of Family Health Services Authorities, Health Authorities and NHS Trusts on important national issues affecting the NHS. In our aim of developing and furthering the interests of health care we aim:

- [ ] to foster co-operation and communication between NHS authorities, government departments, local authorities and other organizations concerned with health matters;
- [ ] to educate and inform the public about the achievements and needs of the NHS;
- [ ] to promote research, education and the exchange of information within the NHS;
- [ ] to advise government and professional bodies on issues relating to the NHS;
- [ ] to investigate specific problems of concern to Family Health Services Authorities, Health Authorities and the newly established NHS Trusts.

NAHAT is financed by its member organizations and generates income.

1 Reforming the NHS

As the NHS enters the 1990s, it is undergoing a programme of reforms more fundamental than any experienced since its inception in 1948. These reforms stem from three White Papers: *Promoting Better Health, Working for Patients, and Caring for People.*

Box 1 The White Papers

Promoting Better Health	1987
Working for Patients	1989
Caring for People	1989

The proposals set out in the White Papers will have a major impact on the delivery of services to patients and the organization and financing of the NHS and local authority community care services. The pages which follow describe the nature of these changes and the implications for NHS authorities.

The Government has emphasized that the basic principles on which the NHS was founded are not affected by its reforms. Health services will continue to be available to all, irrespective of means, on the basis of need. Also, most services will be provided free at the point of use.

Working for Patients

Working for Patients was the outcome of the ministerial review of the NHS. The review was established to address underlying problems in the management and funding of the NHS.

The changes outlined in the White Paper are designed to tackle these problems and to increase the efficiency with which resources are used. The Government also expects that services will become more responsive to users.

These objectives are to be achieved through a number of reforms. The most important of these reforms are:

☐ the introduction of a new system of contractual funding
☐ measures to manage clinical activity more effectively
☐ proposals to strengthen management at all levels
☐ new arrangements for allocating resources.

Contractual Funding

At the heart of the reforms is the idea that there should be a clearer purchasing role within the NHS. This is intended to put hospitals and other provider units under competitive pressure to improve the quality and efficiency of their services. To this end, responsibility for the funding and provision of services is being separated.

In future, the main function of District Health Authorities will be to assess the health of the resident population, determine its health needs, and purchase services to meet these needs. GP practices that serve more than 9,000 patients will also be able to become purchasers of some hospital services if they are accepted as fund-holding practices. Responsibility for service provision will increasingly rest with hospitals and other units. These units will be given more responsibility and some may choose to become NHS Trusts.

NHS contracts or service agreements will be negotiated between health authorities and GP fund-holders as purchasers of care, and hospitals and units (including NHS Trusts) as providers of care. These contracts will specify the quality, quantity, and cost of services to be provided, and they will enable purchasers to hold providers accountable for their performance. There will be three types of contract: cost per case, cost and volume, and block contracts. Disputes or disagreements between purchasers and providers will be resolved locally through the management process.

The introduction of contractual funding will bring about managed competition between provider units. The specification of services in contracts is intended to provide an incentive to ensure that resources go more directly to the hospitals and units which offer the highest quality and best value care. In some cases, NHS hospitals and units

Box 2   Contractual Funding

Separation of funding and provision

NHS Trusts

GP fund-holding practices

Contracts or service agreements

will compete with providers in the voluntary and private sectors for the resources that health authorities and GP fund-holders have to spend.

Units will move towards NHS Trust status gradually. In the immediate future, trusts will operate alongside hospitals and services that remain under the management control of health authorities. The Government has emphasized that the introduction of contractual funding will be carefully managed to ensure that appropriate services continue to be available in each area.

Managing Clinical Activity

A series of measures are being introduced to manage clinical activity more effectively. One important development is the extension of the resource management programme which was established following the Griffiths Report on general management in 1983 (*see* chapter 3). This involves doctors and nurses taking more control over the management of resources and greater responsibility for many of the day-to-day management processes.

There are a variety of ways of achieving this but in many hospitals services are increasingly run by clinical directors (usually doctors) with support from a nurse manager and often from a business manager. These staff have a budget to run their service and these budgets are linked to work-load agreements negotiated with the hospital manager. At the same time, information systems are being developed to provide staff with better data about the services they deliver.

Until recently, resource management operated in six acute hospital sites. It is now being extended rapidly, with all large acute hospitals able to join the programme by March 1992.

Box 3 Managing Clinical Activity

Resource management programme

PACT data for GPs

Medical audit

Managers to be involved in consultants' appointments

Managers to agree job plans with consultants

Managers to participate in decisions on distinction awards

New disciplinary procedures

GPs are also being provided with better tools and support. This includes prescribing, analysis, and cost (PACT) data to enable them to monitor prescribing patterns. Medical advisers to Family Health Services Authorities (FHSAs) review clinical issues with GPs, including referral patterns.

Medical audit is being introduced in both hospitals and primary care. Audit involves doctors reviewing their clinical practices systematically with colleagues to identify areas in which improvements can be made. District Health Authorities, NHS Trusts, and Family Health Services Authorities will be expected to set up medical audit advisory committees to ensure that effective arrangements for audit are in place.

The Government is also expecting general managers to play a bigger part in the management of clinical activity. In future, managers will participate in the appointment of consultants, and they will agree a job plan with each consultant. To emphasize the clinician's role in management, the criteria for distinction awards have been modified to include a commitment on the part of consultants to the management of services. A general manager will be involved in decisions about which consultants receive distinction awards.

The other major change is the introduction of new disciplinary procedures for hospital doctors. These procedures will enable disciplinary matters to be dealt with more expeditiously.

Better Management

A theme running through the reforms is the need to introduce better management at all levels. In the Department of Health (DoH), this has been achieved through the establishment of the Policy Board, chaired by the Secretary of State, and the Management Executive, chaired by the NHS Chief Executive. The Policy Board and the NHS Management Executive are intended to provide clearer leadership of the NHS at the centre.

In the NHS, the role of District Health Authorities will change, and will increasingly focus on identifying health needs and purchasing services to meet needs. Family Health Services Authorities' key tasks will be to assess the need for primary health care services of their residents and ensure that these services are provided by family doctors, dentists, pharmacists, and opticians. In so doing, they will operate through the terms of the contracts negotiated nationally with family practitioners.

Box 4   Better Management

Policy Board and Management Executive

New role of NHS authorities

New membership of NHS authorities

Devolution of decision-making

Regional Health Authorities (RHAs) and District Health Authorities will have a revised membership. This involves members from outside coming together with key officers into smaller bodies comprising executive and non-executive members and a chairman. Family Health Services Authorities have also been streamlined and will comprise the general manager, the chairman, and nine non-executive members (including four professionals).

A strong emphasis has been placed on the devolution of decision-making. As far as possible, those who provide services will have the power to take decisions about operational matters.

Allocating Resources

A number of changes will be made to the way in which resources are allocated. GPs who are eligible and who are accepted will receive a practice fund from the Regional Health Authority to buy a defined range of services for their patients. These services comprise out-patients' services, diagnostic tests, and in-patient and day-care treatments for which there is some choice over the time and place of treatment. The cost of these services will be deducted from the allocation of the relevant District Health Authority. The practice fund will also include an amount to cover the cost of prescribing. Family Health Services Authorities will monitor expenditure against the fund.

GPs who are not in fund-holding practices will have indicative prescribing amounts (formerly known as budgets). This is part of a policy of improving the efficiency, quality, and value for money of drug prescribing. Family Health Services Authorities will set and monitor prescribing amounts and will also allocate development funds for GP staff and premises.

Box 5 Allocating Resources

GPs to purchase some hospital services

Indicative prescribing amounts

Family Health Services Authorities to allocate funds for GP staff and premises

District Health Authorities funded as purchasers not providers

Money follows patients

Capital charges

Significant changes are being made to the allocation of resources to District Health Authorities. In future, District Health Authorities will receive funds to purchase services for their residents instead of being allocated funds to provide services in their hospitals. This means a shift from funding health authorities as *providers* of health services to funding them as *purchasers* of health services. Allocations will be made on a weighted capitation basis.

The resources received by District Health Authorities will not be adjusted for the flow of patients across boundaries. Instead, authorities will pay for their residents to be treated outside their districts through the contracts that are negotiated with providers. In this way, money will follow patients. The establishment of a funding system for hospitals in which money follows patients is intended to create a stronger incentive for hospitals to treat people as consumers and to agree contracts with purchasers.

Another key change is the introduction of a new system of charging for capital. This will require hospitals to recognize capital costs (depreciation and interest) in respect of the assets that they use. The aim of capital charges is to stimulate managers to use capital assets more efficiently. Capital charges will also allow the costs of NHS provision to be evaluated on a basis broadly comparable with the private sector.

Promoting Better Health

The second area in which reform is occurring is primary health care. The Government set out its proposals for change in a consultative document issued in 1986. A period of wide consultation led to the publication of the White Paper *Promoting Better Health* in 1987.

The main aims of the primary care reforms are to raise standards of health and health care, to place greater emphasis on health promotion and disease prevention, and to offer wider choice and information to patients. Many of these reforms were introduced through the contracts under which family doctors and dentists provide services. A new contract for GPs came into effect on 1 April 1990 and for dentists on 1 October 1990.

In the case of GPs, the contract includes provision for health checks for new patients, three-yearly checks for patients not otherwise seen by a GP, and annual checks for patients aged 75 and over. In parallel, targets have been set for vaccination, immunization, and cervical cancer screening, encouragement has been given to the development of health promotion clinics and the provision of minor surgery, and GPs will be expected to become more closely involved in child health surveillance.

Other features of the new contract include extra payments for doctors practising in deprived areas, additional money to employ practice staff and improve practice premises, and a requirement that practices produce an annual report and information leaflets for patients. The procedure through which patients change their doctor has also been simplified.

Box 6 *Promoting Better Health*

New contracts for doctors and dentists

Raised standards of care

Emphasis on health promotion and disease prevention

Information and choice for patients

In the case of family dentists, the new contract emphasizes the need for dental care to include preventive work as well as restorative treatments. Regular patients will be entitled to:

☐ more information about their treatment in a treatment plan
☐ emergency cover arrangements
☐ replacement free of charge for certain restorations which fail within a year for adults.

As far as children are concerned, dentists will receive a capitation payment for each child instead of being paid by item of service for treatment given. Also, all patients will receive more information about dental services. Part of the cost of these changes has been met by the removal of most adult eye tests from the NHS and the introduction of a charge for adult dental examinations.

The various reforms stemming from *Promoting Better Health* are reinforced by the changes outlined in *Working for Patients*. As highlighted in the previous section, these changes include:

☐ arrangements to enable larger practices to hold funds to purchase certain hospital services
☐ the introduction of the indicative prescribing scheme for other GPs
☐ the development of medical audit.

8

Family Health Services Authorities will pay a key part in implementing these changes. To assist them in this process, Family Health Services Authorities have recently appointed general managers, and their membership has been reconstituted in line with their management responsibilities.

Caring for People

The White Paper *Caring for People* was the Government's response to the Griffiths Report, *Community Care: Agenda for Action*, published in 1988.

The White Paper seeks to overcome the slow and uneven development of services across the country by giving local authorities the lead responsibility in the planning of community care. Local authorities will be expected to review the need for care in their areas, develop community care plans in association with NHS authorities and other agencies, and secure the provision of relevant services. Some of these services may be provided directly by local authorities but increasingly they will become enablers and purchasers, co-ordinating the provision of care in the public, private, and voluntary sectors.

These changes go hand in hand with new funding arrangements. Expenditure on residential care through the social security budget has increased from £10 million in 1979 to £1,000 million in 1989. One of the main purposes of the reforms is to ensure that the money involved is correctly targeted and spent effectively.

Under the new arrangements, the income support available to people in need of assistance from public funds and paid under social security provisions will be the same whether they live at home or in voluntary or private sector residential care. In addition, some of the money that has previously been allocated through the social security budget will be transferred to local authorities to enable them to purchase care. The aim of this change is to remove the incentive that has existed in the past to admit people to private and voluntary residential accommodation with the bill being paid by the Department of Social Security (DSS).

The Government intends that local authorities should use the new funding arrangements to develop more effective domiciliary care. This includes practical support for carers. Assessment of an individual's care needs will be a cornerstone of the new arrangements along with case management systems to secure the most appropriate packages of care.

The Government expects the voluntary and private sectors to play a bigger part in service provision. Local authorities will set up independent inspection units to monitor the quality of care, initially in residential provision.

Box 7 *Caring for People*

> Local authorities to have lead responsibility
>
> Local authorities as enablers and purchasers
>
> Community care plans
>
> New funding arrangements
>
> Support for domiciliary care and carers
>
> Assessment and case management
>
> Independent inspection units
>
> Collaboration with NHS authorities

The success of these changes hinges on effective collaboration between local authorities, District Health Authorities, and Family Health Services Authorities. If a co-ordinated approach is not developed, it will be difficult to provide the seamless service needed by those requiring care and support.

Implementation of the community care reforms is taking place over a three-year period.

Summary

Many of the changes discussed in this section are enshrined in the NHS and Community Care Act 1990. The Act gives the Government the legal powers necessary to implement *Working for Patients* and

Caring for People. Its provisions are being implemented at a steady pace and will provide for further developments in coming years.

The programme of reforms on which the Government has embarked represents a major challenge for NHS authorities and trusts and local authorities. Although the broad framework has been established at a national level, much depends on the ability and imagination of those responsible for implementing the reforms locally. The new areas of responsibility included in the legislation create an opportunity to improve local health and community care services and to tackle long-standing weaknesses in service delivery.

Further Reading

Secretary of State for Health and others (1989), *Working for Patients*, HMSO, London.

Secretary of State for Social Services and others (1987), *Promoting Better Health*, HMSO, London.

Secretary of State for Health and others (1989), *Caring for People*, HMSO, London.

King's Fund Institute (1989), *Managed Competition*, London.

Working Paper No. 1 (1989), *Self-governing Hospitals*, HMSO, London.

Working Paper No. 2 (1989), *Funding and Contracts for Hospital Services*, HMSO, London.

Working Paper No. 3 (1989), *Practice Budgets for General Medical Practitioners*, HMSO, London.

Working Paper No. 4 (1989), *Indicative Prescribing Budgets for General Medical Practitioners*, HMSO, London.

Working Paper No. 5 (1989), *Capital Charges*, HMSO, London.

Working Paper No. 6 (1989), *Medical Audit*, HMSO, London.

Working Paper No. 7 (1989), *NHS Consultants: Appointments, Contracts and Distinction Awards*, HMSO, London.

Working Paper No. 8 (1989), *Implications for Family Practitioner Committees*, HMSO, London.

Working Paper No. 9 (1989), *Capital Charges: Funding Issues*, HMSO, London.

Working Paper No. 10 (1989), *Education and Training*, HMSO, London.

Working Paper No. 11 (1990), *Framework for Information Systems: Overview*, HMSO, London.

Self-governing Hospitals: An initial guide, HMSO, London.

Role of District Health Authorities – Analysis of Issues, HMSO, London.

Developing Districts, (1990), Department of Health, London.

Improving Prescribing, (1990), Department of Health, London.

(1989), *Funding General Practice*, Department of Health, London.
National Association of Health Authorities and Trusts Briefing No. 2 (1990), *The National Health Service and Community Care Act 1990*, Birmingham.

2 The Organization of the NHS

The organization of the NHS in England is illustrated in Figure 1. Differences in the rest of the UK are outlined at the end of this chapter.

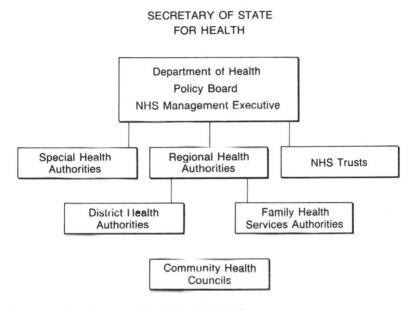

Figure 1. Organization of the NHS in England.

The Secretary of State for Health is responsible to Parliament for the provision of health services. The Secretary of State discharges his responsibility through Regional Health Authorities, District Health Authorities, Family Health Services Authorities, NHS Trusts, and Special Health Authorities (SHAs). Community Health Councils (CHCs) are statutory bodies established at a local level to represent the interests of their communities in the NHS, but lie outside the managerial chain.

The Department of Health

The Department of Health is responsible at a national level for the NHS and also for setting the policy and legislative framework for the personal social services and other health issues. The Secretary of State for Health sits at the head of the Department and he is supported by a Minister of State for Health and by a number of junior ministers. Some 5,200 civil servants work in the Department. The most senior of these civil servants are the Permanent Secretary, the Chief Medical Officer (CMO), and the Chief Executive of the NHS Management Executive.

The Secretary of State is assisted within the Department on NHS matters by the Policy Board and the Management Executive. The Policy Board sets the broad strategic direction for the NHS and the Management Executive deals with all operational matters within the strategy and objectives established by the Policy Board. The Policy Board is chaired by the Secretary of State and its members include a number of businessmen, people drawn from the NHS, officials (including the Permanent Secretary and Chief Executive), and health ministers. The Management Executive is chaired by the Chief Executive of the NHS and its members comprise civil servants and people from business and the NHS.

The Department of Health performs a number of functions in relation to the NHS. Policy and advice are issued in various forms. Major policy statements are usually set out in White Papers or discussion documents. Detailed advice and guidance is issued through health circulars, health notices, and executive letters.

Box 8 Functions of the Department of Health on NHS Matters

Making policy and issuing advice to authorities
Allocating resources
Monitoring the performance of authorities and holding them to account

Resources are allocated annually following the negotiations which take place in the Government's Public Expenditure Survey. It is through the Survey that priorities for different areas of public spending are determined.

The outcome of the Survey is announced in the Chancellor's Autumn Statement to Parliament and detailed information about each public expenditure programme is given in the annual Public Expenditure White Paper (PEWP). From January 1991 the Public Expenditure White Paper will be replaced by a series of individual Departmental Reports. These will continue to fulfil the same functions as the Public Expenditure White Paper in terms of accounting for public expenditure.

The Department of Health retains some resources to run its own operations and allocates funds to the Special Health Authorities (*see* below), but the great bulk of the health service budget is distributed to Regional Health Authorities. In future, the resources received by Regional Health Authorities will be used by District Health Authorities to purchase hospital and community health services and by Family Health Services Authorities to pay for the family health services. Separate allocations are made for revenue and capital expenditure (*see* chapter 4 for more details of finance).

The Department of Health monitors the performance of NHS authorities and assesses the way in which they use resources through the review process. This involves continuing discussion between members of the Management Executive and their regional counterparts. The culmination of this process is the formal review meeting between the Chief Executive of the NHS and each regional general manager, supported by their senior colleagues.

The content of the review process, based on the region's agreed objectives, includes both service and management issues. Some issues will be discussed with all regions (e.g. waiting-lists and waiting-times), others will be specific to individual regions. In turn, Regional Health Authorities review the performance of District Health Authorities and Family Health Services Authorities. The cycle is completed when District Health Authorities review the performance of their directly managed units and Family Health Services Authorities monitor the performance of family practitioners.

The emphasis of reviews is increasingly on looking forward as well as back, including discussion of the Regional Health Authority's major objectives for the coming financial year.

Parliamentary Accountability

The NHS is financed almost entirely from public funds. Parliament votes £22 billion per annum for the NHS in England and expects some say in how that money is spent. The accountability of the Secretary of State to Parliament has an important bearing on the organization and management of the NHS.

Individual MPs are able to raise issues in correspondence and through parliamentary questions and debates, and the Secretary of State is expected to be able to respond to these issues. In so doing, the Secretary of State through his civil servants may ask NHS authorities to supply information and advice, often at short notice. Parliamentary accountability thus acts as a centralizing influence in the NHS.

The Public Accounts Committee of the House of Commons examines the NHS from time to time, paying particular attention to the way in which the money voted by Parliament has been spent. The Committee is supported in its work by the Comptroller and Auditor General and the National Audit Office (NAO). The National Audit Office carries out studies into particular aspects of the NHS and these studies are used by the Public Accounts Committee as a basis for its enquiries. The Chief Executive of the Management Executive is the Accounting Officer for most aspects of the NHS and is called before the Committee as required to give evidence and answer questions.

The Health Committee (one of the successors of the Social Services Committee) is one of a number of Departmental select committees and its job is to investigate the work of the Department of Health. The Committee takes oral and written evidence from ministers, civil servants, and others involved in health policy and the provision of health services. It will take forward the work of the Social Services Committee in producing reports on issues such as the reform of the NHS and the Government's expenditure plans and priorities.

The Structure of the Department of Health

The responsibilities of the Department of Health cover three distinct businesses: health, health care, and social services. Each business has its own management chain and executive agencies. The business structure of the Department is illustrated in Figure 2.

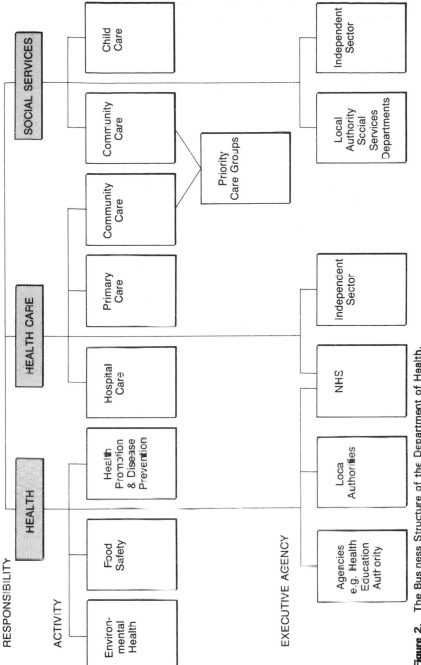

Figure 2. The Business Structure of the Department of Health.

As far as the health care business is concerned, the Department's work is organized in broad terms into three main areas. Health care policy comes under the Health and Social Services Divisions (formerly known as the Policy Group). The management of the NHS comes under the NHS Management Executive and its Divisions. Both policy and management draw on common services such as analytical support from the Central Resource Management Divisions. The three sets of Divisions interlock and, for example, issues that involve both policy and management considerations are handled through joint working between the Health and Social Services Divisions and the Management Executive. The tripartite structure is illustrated in Figure 3.

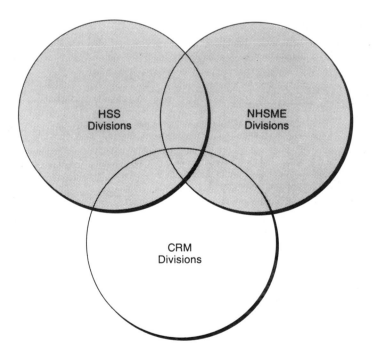

Figure 3. The Tripartite Structure.

It is important to emphasize that the perspective of civil servants may be different from that of NHS authorities and their managers. Departmental officials have a primary duty to support ministers and to promote national policies and objectives. NHS authorities are much more concerned with local issues and the challenge of purchasing and providing services on a day-to-day basis. The two perspectives may not always point in the same direction and each side may feel that its position is not appreciated by the other.

In recent years there has been increasing interchange of personnel between the Department of Health and the NHS. Civil servants have been seconded to work in NHS authorities and some have moved to the NHS on a permanent basis. Equally, a number of NHS staff have been brought in to work in the Department. These exchanges help in building understanding and mutual respect, and there are plans to make greater use of secondments in the future.

Formal contact and communication between the Department and the NHS is maintained in a number of other ways. These include:

☐ regular meetings between ministers and Regional Health Authority chairmen and between civil servants and the staff of authorities
☐ joint working between the Department and the NHS through working parties and advisory groups
☐ discussions between the Department and representative national groups such as the National Association of Health Authorities and Trusts, and the Institute of Health Services Management.

Within the Department the Regional Liaison Division in the Management Executive is a key point of contact for NHS authorities. The regional principal for each Regional Health Authority acts as a two-way channel of communication between the Department and authorities. In parallel, the NHS Trusts unit in the Management Executive acts as the link between trusts and the Department.

Regional Health Authorities

Regional Health Authorities are the intermediate tier between the Department of Health on the one hand and District Health Authorities and Family Health Services Authorities on the other. There are 14 Regional Health Authorities in England serving populations ranging from 2 million to over 5 million (*see* Figure 4, page 22). The revenue budget of Regional Health Authorities varies from £558 million to £1,458 million.

Each authority comprises a chairman and five non-executive members appointed by the Secretary of State together with up to five executive members. Two of the executives, the general manager and chief finance officer, are ex-officio members. The remainder are appointed by the chairman and non-executive members together with the general manager. The Regional Health Authority works as a corporate body and is accountable to the Secretary of State.

Regional Health Authorities perform a number of functions in the NHS. These are mainly concerned with planning, resource allocation, and monitoring performance. Regional Health Authorities also have a significant part to play in implementing the Government's reforms of the NHS. This includes guiding the introduction of NHS Trusts, overseeing implementation of new funding systems for GPs and NHS authorities, leading the development of contracting, and ensuring that District Health Authorities and Family Health Services Authorities introduce the reforms on time and in a managed way.

Box 9   The Functions of Regional Health Authorities

Planning the development of services within the context of national guidelines

Allocating resources to District Health Authorities, Family Health Services Authorities, and GP fund-holders

Monitoring the performance of District Health Authorities and Family Health Services Authorities and holding them to account

---

To enable them to concentrate on key strategic tasks, regions have recently reviewed the provision of their directly managed and operational services. These services have been retained at regional level only if they are essential to the responsibilities of Regional Health Authorities or if District Health Authorities wish Regional Health Authorities to retain a role in service provision.

Regional Health Authorities will continue to play a part in managing the capital building programme (except for NHS Trusts), and they will also act as the establishing authority for Community Health Councils. A further responsibility is to appoint the non-executive members of District Health Authorities and Family Health Services Authorities and two of the non-executive directors of NHS Trusts.

Regional Health Authorities will take on new responsibilities in three areas. The first concerns family health services. In future, Family Health Authorities will be held accountable to Regional Health Authorities instead of directly to the Department of Health. To help build understanding between the two kinds of authority, each Regional Health Authority includes a Family Health Services Authority chairman among its non-executive members.

The second responsibility new to Regional Health Authorities is regulation of the relationship between purchasers and providers. If there are disputes between purchasers and providers, then Regional Health Authorities will provide a conciliation service. They will also have a broader responsibility to ensure that managed competition does not undermine the availability and accessibility of services or distort priorities in service provision.

Thirdly, Regional Health Authorites have been given responsibility for the planning and funding of education and training for non-medical staff. This includes assessing demand and ensuring that there is an adequate supply of staff.

Regional Health Authorities thus have a key role in the NHS. The responsibilities of regions have steadily increased during the 1980s and the NHS reforms take this a stage further. It is clearly not practical for the Department of Health to manage District Health Authorities and Family Health Services Authorities directly. For the foreseeable future, Regional Health Authorities will be expected to act on behalf of the Department in planning and managing services in their localities.

District Health Authorities

District Health Authorities are the bodies responsible for purchasing hospital and community health services for their residents. There are

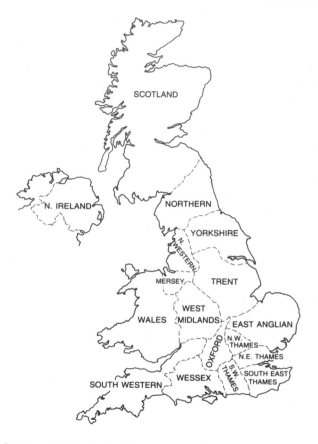

Figure 4. Regional Health Authorities.

189 District Health Authorities in England with populations ranging from 89,000 to 860,000. The revenue budget varies from £13 million to £183 million.

Each authority comprises a chairman appointed by the Secretary of State, five non-executive members appointed by the Regional Health Authority, and up to five executive members. Two of the executives, the general manager and the chief finance officer, are ex-officio members. The remainder are appointed by the chairman and non-executive members together with the general manager. The District

Health Authority works as a corporate body and is accountable to the Regional Health Authority.

District Health Authorities perform a number of functions in the NHS. These include purchasing health care for their residents and managing the services provided in directly managed units (DMUs). District Health Authorities also have a number of traditional public health responsibilities. As the role of District Health Authorities develops, they will assess the population's need for health care.

In deciding which services to purchase, District Health Authorities are expected to work closely with Family Health Services Authorities, GPs, local authorities, and other agencies to build up an assessment of the health state of their population. They will also consult health service users and their representatives. When NHS Trusts are set up, trusts will assume responsibility for service provision. District Health Authorities will, however, continue to manage the units which remain under their control until such time as those units become NHS Trusts.

Box 10   Functions of District Health Authorities

Purchasing services for their residents
Managing units which remain under their control
Assessing the population's need for health care
Public health

These directly managed units will be given greater autonomy within the framework set by the District Health Authority and the contracts under which they operate. The implication of these changes is that District Health Authorities will devolve responsibility for operational decision-making to directly managed units. Many functions which have been previously carried out at district level, such as personnel, finance, and information services, will be transferred to units, although some may be organized on a common services basis.

As a consequence, district staff will focus on their new purchasing role. This means bringing together a core group of staff with expertise in public health, contracting, and quality assurance to work with the general manager and chief finance officer. As these changes are implemented, District Health Authorities will become leaner, slimmer bodies responsible for taking a strategic view of health needs and securing services to meet these needs.

Family Health Services Authorities

Family Health Services Authorities manage the services provided by general medical practitioners, general dental practitioners, retail pharmacists, and opticians. These family practitioners are independent contractors and are not employees of the NHS. The terms and conditions under which family practitioners work in the NHS are negotiated nationally and Family Health Services Authorities are responsible for implementing the national contracts in their area.

There are 90 Family Health Services Authorities in England serving populations ranging from about 130,000 to 1,600,000. Each conforms to a major local authority area and generally follows the geographical boundaries of District Health Authorities. Some 37 Family Health Services Authorities relate to one District Health Authority, with the balance relating to anything from two to seven District Health Authorities.

Each authority comprises a chairman appointed by the Secretary of State, five lay non-executive members and four professional non-executives (a GP, dentist, pharmacist, and community nurse) appointed by the Regional Health Authority. The authority also includes a general manager appointed by the chairman and non-executive members. The Family Health Services Authority works as a corporate body and is accountable as an authority to the Regional Health Authority.

Family Health Services Authorities perform a number of functions. These include managing the contracts of family practitioners, paying practitioners in accordance with contracts, providing information to the public, and dealing with complaints made by patients.

Box 11   The Functions of Family Health Services Authorities

Managing the contracts of family practitioners

Assessing the population's need for health care

Planning services to meet those needs

Managing GP development funds

Family Health Services Authorities are also responsible for planning and developing services in order to meet the health needs of the population. This function will become more important as a consequence of the Government's NHS reforms. In particular, Family Health Services Authorities will be expected to:

☐ assess the health needs of the population
☐ develop services to meet those needs
☐ ensure that quality services are provided efficiently and cost-effectively.

One of the ways in which they will pursue these objectives is through the management of funds for GP practice developments. Control over these funds, which cover practice staff and improvements to premises, will enable Family Health Services Authorities to target resources where they are most needed.

In carrying out their responsibilities, Family Health Services Authorities will need to develop an information base for planning purposes, establish criteria for allocating the resources at their disposal, and work closely with other agencies such as District Health Authorities and local authorities.

They will also take on a number of new functions. These include carrying out consumer surveys, introducing medical audit, setting up and monitoring indicative prescribing amounts, working with Regional Health Authorities on the introduction of GP fund-holding and monitoring the operation of the new dental contract. These tasks, along with established responsibilities in areas such as approving surgery locations and hours of availability, checking the standard of premises, and authorizing and monitoring the use of deputizing services, amount to a significant programme of work.

25

NHS Trusts

Hospitals and other units providing patient care may be established as NHS Trusts. These are 'self-governing' units within the NHS. They are run by boards of directors and are accountable directly to the Secretary of State without any intervention from District or Regional Health Authorities.

Trusts will have individual functions and will have a range of freedoms not available to units remaining under district management. In particular they will be free to determine their own management structures, to employ their own staff and set their own terms and conditions of service, to acquire, own, and sell their own assets, to retain surpluses, and to borrow money subject to annual limits.

Each Trust will be required to prepare an annual business plan outlining, among other things, its plans for service development and capital investment. These plans will be discussed with the NHS Management Executive but will not be public documents. Each Trust will also prepare and publish an annual report and accounts.

Like other units, Trusts will receive their income from contracts with health authorities, GP fund-holders, and other purchasers. They will be responsible to purchasers for delivering the quantity and quality of care specified in these contracts.

The underlying aim of establishing Trusts is to improve the quality of care provided to patients by giving real power and responsibility to those people – managers, doctors, nurses, and other staff – who work in the unit and by harnessing their skills and commitment for the benefit of patient care.

Special Health Authorities

Some NHS services are administered by Special Health Authorities responsible for certain areas of activity. Examples are the eight authorities covering London's postgraduate teaching hospitals, the Health Education Authority (HEA), the Mental Health Act Commission, the NHS Training Authority (NHSTA), and the Special Hospitals Service Authority. The Special Health Authorities are not part of the NHS structure but are directly accountable to the Secretary of State.

Community Health Councils

Community Health Councils are statutory bodies established by Regional Health Authorities to represent the public interest in the local provision of health services and to be the channel for consumer concerns. As a general rule, there is one Community Health Council for every District Health Authority.

Community Health Councils normally have 18 to 24 members. One third are nominated by voluntary organizations, one half are nominated by local authorities, and one sixth are nominated by the Regional Health Authority. The Secretary of the Community Health Council is a paid employee of the Regional Health Authority, appointed by the Regional Health Authority in consultation with the Community Health Council. Most Community Health Councils operate on an annual budget of £35,000 – 40,000 provided by the Regional Health Authority.

Community Health Councils are one of the channels through which the public's voice is heard in the NHS. In order to support them in their role, Parliament has agreed that Community Health Councils should have the following rights:

☐ to relevant information from local NHS authorities
☐ to access to certain NHS premises
☐ to inclusion in consultation on substantial developments or variations in service
☐ to send observers to meetings of matching District Health Authorities and Family Health Services Authorities.

Community Health Councils have a duty to publish an annual report and this is discussed at meetings with the District Health Authority and Family Health Services Authority. Community Health Councils have few formal powers and in the main have to seek to influence decisions through advice, information, and persuasion.

Wales, Scotland and Northern Ireland

There are important differences in the organization of health services in Wales, Scotland and Northern Ireland. Responsibility for health

27

services in these countries rests with the Welsh Office, the Scottish Office, and the Northern Ireland Office respectively. There is no regional tier of management. Functions which are the responsibility of Regional Health Authorities in England are performed either by the health departments at national level or by local health authorities. There are also common services agencies in areas where it is cost-effective to provide services nationally.

At a local level, health services in Wales are organized through nine District Health Authorities and eight Family Health Services Authorities. In Scotland, there are 15 Health Boards and these boards are responsible for family health services as well as hospital and community health services. In Northern Ireland, there are four Health and Social Services Boards. As their name indicates, these boards cover personal social services as well as hospital and community health services and family health services.

The public's interest in the NHS is represented by Community Health Councils in Wales, Local Health Councils in Scotland, and District Committees in Northern Ireland.

Further Reading

Secretary of State for Health and others (1989), *Working for Patients*, HMSO, London.

3 | Managing Health Services

The management of the NHS has undergone a series of changes in recent years. The Griffiths Report of 1983 led to the appointment of general managers; *Working for Patients* has resulted in major changes to the composition and role of NHS authorities; and a variety of initiatives have put the quality of services high on the management agenda. In this section we review these developments and examine their implications for the NHS.

General Management

In 1983 a team led by Sir Roy Griffiths, managing director and deputy chairman of the retailers Sainsbury's, produced a report on health services management. The Griffiths Report was highly critical of management at all levels in the NHS. At the centre, it found that the Department of Health did not provide effective leadership of the NHS; in the case of health authorities, it criticized the system of consensus management through multidisciplinary teams for failing to deliver the drive and imagination needed in a modern health service; and the report also argued that within hospitals doctors should play a much bigger part in management.

Box 12 Extracts from the Griffiths Report

'One of our most immediate observations from a business background is the lack of a clearly defined general management function throughout the NHS. By general management we mean the responsibility drawn together in one person, at different levels of the organization, for planning, implementation, and control of performance.'

'Absence of this general management support means that there is no driving force seeking and accepting direct and personal responsibility for developing management plans, securing their implementation, and monitoring actual achievement.'

continued overleaf

Box 12 *continued*

> 'The centre is still too much involved in too many of the wrong things and too little involved in some that really matter.'
>
> 'To the outsider, it appears that when change of any kind is required, the NHS is so structured as to resemble a "mobile" designed to move with any breath of air, but which in fact never changes its position and gives no clear indication of direction.'
>
> 'The nearer that the management process gets to the patient, the more important it becomes for the doctors to be looked upon as the natural managers.'
>
> 'Action is now badly needed and the health service can ill afford to indulge in any lengthy self-imposed Hamlet-like soliloquy as a precursor or alternative to the required action.'

The Secretary of State accepted the findings of the Griffiths Report and announced that its recommendations would be implemented.

As a consequence general managers were introduced at regional, district, and unit levels, accountable for the total performance of their organization. Management systems were refined and developed, including the introduction of performance-related pay and individual performance review. Both were later extended to other management levels. The employment package for general managers also included short-term (usually three-year) rolling contracts. The intention of these changes was to place a high premium on achieving improvements in services and to break away from the inertia that was sometimes a feature of consensus management.

Box 13 The Introduction of General Management

> The appointment of general managers at all levels
>
> Short-term contracts for general managers
>
> Individual performance review
>
> Performance-related pay

The introduction of general management had a number of other effects. In place of management teams which had the same membership everywhere, a variety of management arrangements emerged to suit local circumstances. This included the appointment of senior managers to take responsibility for quality assurance as part of the move to make services more responsive to consumers.

Another effect was to devolve decision-making powers from District Health Authorities to units of management. Devolution did not occur universally, but where it did units were given more responsibility to manage services within parameters and objectives set by the District Health Authority.

In parallel with these changes, the NHS Management Board (the forerunner of the Management Executive) pioneered the introduction of management budgeting and its successor, the resource management programme. In broad terms, resource management seeks to improve patient care by:

- giving doctors and nurses a bigger role in the management of resources
- devolving budgetary responsibility to clinical teams within hospitals
- enabling managers to negotiate work-load agreements with these clinical teams
- improving information systems to provide staff with better data about their services.

Initially resource management was developed at six acute hospital sites where medical and nursing staff were known to support the principles involved.

Box 14   The Six Acute Pilot Sites

Arrowe Park Hospital, Wirral
Freeman Hospital, Newcastle
Guy's Hospital, London
The Royal Hampshire County Hospital, Winchester
The Royal Infirmary, Huddersfield
The Pilgrim Hospital, Lincolnshire

Following promising progress reports from the six sites, and the ministerial review of the NHS, the Government decided to extend resource management rapidly to other hospitals. Central funds were set aside to support implementation and a heavy emphasis was placed on training and organizational development.

Human Resources

The Griffiths Report emphasized the need to manage human resources more effectively within the NHS. In particular, the Report recommended that the Whitley Council system for agreeing pay and conditions of service at a national level should be reviewed to examine whether greater devolution was possible. This recommendation was echoed by *Working for Patients* which stated that the Government's objective was to introduce flexibility to allow managers to relate pay rates to local labour markets and to reward individual performance.

The emphasis placed on the effective management of human resources is not surprising as the NHS is a major employer. Figure 5 illustrates the distribution of staff (totalling 793,000 in England in 1988) between different occupational groups.

A particular concern of NHS authorities and Trusts at present is the difficulty likely to be experienced in recruiting staff in the 1990s. This is because of a shortfall in the number of school leavers coupled with increased competition for staff from higher education and the service sector. Various strategies are being pursued in tackling this difficulty including more flexible working arrangements and pay systems, attempts to retain staff already in post, offering child care, and encouraging women to return to work after a career break.

Staff training and development in the NHS takes a number of forms. In the case of nurses, the single biggest group of employees, major changes are taking place, based on the Project 2000 report prepared by the United Kingdom Central Council (UKCC) for nursing, midwifery and health visitors. Project 2000 students will receive a bursary rather than a salary, and will be supernumary for most of their clinical placements. They will qualify as registered nurses in one of four branches: general nursing of adults, mental health nursing, mental handicap nursing, and children's nursing. Enrolled nurse training is being phased out.

32

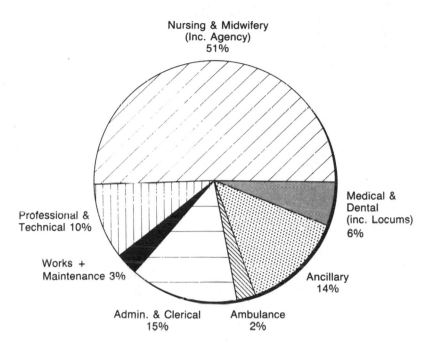

Figure 5. NHS Directly Employed Staff by Main Staff Group, England, 1988.

The NHS Training Authority is concerned with the development of managers and other occupational groups in the NHS. It does not involve itself in professional training where this is the responsibility of another professional or statutory body. In 1986 the NHS Training Authority published *Better Management, Better Health* setting out its policy for management development in the NHS. Among other things, this led to the introduction of individual performance review for general managers (*see* page 30) and the general management training scheme. More recently, priority has been given to the training of middle managers.

NHS authorities and Trusts are responsible as employers for deciding local personnel policies. These policies encompass issues such as:

☐ industrial relations
☐ equal opportunities

☐ health and safety at work
☐ manpower planning and utilization
☐ recruitment and retention of staff
☐ communications, morale and motivation
☐ training and development.

The current national agreements on grievance and disciplinary procedures include rights for staff to appeal (for example on grading) either to a committee of members or in some cases to the full authority.

As in other areas of management, a key objective of the NHS Management Executive is that personnel responsibilities should be exercised as close as possible to the operational level. This implies a substantial strengthening of both specialist personnel management, and the personnel skills of line managers in provider units. Few if any functions will be retained at district level.

The development of a strong personnel function will be particularly important for NHS Trusts which will both employ their own staff and be free to set the terms and conditions of service for such staff without being bound by national agreements. Their task will be made more complex because those staff who transfer to a Trust retain their existing terms and conditions of service unless and until changes are negotiated. At least initially, therefore, Trusts will have some employees on national terms and conditions and others on locally determined terms and conditions.

The Role of NHS Authorities

Under the changes brought about by *Working for Patients* and the NHS and Community Care Act, managers will become members of authorities for the first time. In Regional Health Authorities and District Health Authorities the chairman works with five non-executive members and up to five executive members. In the case of Family Health Services Authorities, the chairman is joined by nine non-executive members and the general manager. (Throughout this section the term 'members' is used to describe both executives and non-executives who sit on authorities.)

The members of NHS authorities are equal in status and carry corporate responsibility for the work that is done in their name. In

Box 15 The Composition of the New Authorities

	Family Health Services Authority	Regional Health Authority	District Health Authority	NHS Trust
Chairman appointed by	Secretary of State	Secretary of State	Secretary of State	Secretary of State
Non-executives on the authority	Five lay members appointed by Regional Health Authority, four professional members appointed by Regional Health Authority	Five appointed by Secretary of State including a Family Health Services Authority chairman and a member who holds a post in a university with a medical or dental school	Five appointed by Regional Health Authority. Teaching districts to include a member who holds a post in a university with a medical or dental school	Up to five including at least two appointed from local community by Regional Health Authority. Rest to be appointed by Secreatry of State including a person from the relevant medical school where a trust has teaching responsibilities
Executives on the authority	Chief executive	Up to five including chief executive and finance director	Up to five including chief executive and finance director	Up to five including chief executive, finance director, medical director, senior nurse

practice, the chairman's role in leading the authority means that he or she is first among equals. Chairmen have a particular responsibility to ensure that the work of authorities is properly organized and that executive members and non-executive members operate together as a team.

More specifically, chairmen perform a number of functions. These include focusing the attention of authorities on corporate aims and strategy, controlling authority meetings, making sure the time available is used constructively, and representing the authority to higher levels of management. Chairmen work closely with general managers in carrying out these functions and in guiding the business of authorities. Developing an effective partnership between chairmen and general managers is of the utmost importance.

Day-to-day management responsibility rests with the general manager and his senior colleagues. The decision to allocate places on authorities (initially a single place in the case of Family Health Services Authorities) to managers symbolizes the importance the Government attaches to effective management. Top managers will participate in making the decisions they have to implement and they will play an active part in determining strategies and setting priorities. Ensuring that high-quality managers are appointed is one of the main responsibilities of the chairman and the non-executive members.

Non-executives contribute to the work of authorities in other ways. At one level, their role is to bring independence and detachment, offering a broader perspective than is available through the executive members. At another level, they are responsible for holding the executives to account and for questioning and challenging the advice they receive. Although not appointed in a representative capacity, non-executives act on behalf of the people they serve, making sure that services are managed in a way which is in the interests of the local community.

As corporate bodies, authorities are responsible for establishing overall policy direction and providing leadership for their part of the NHS. In carrying out this responsibility they have to take account of national policies and local needs. Authorities must also operate within resource constraints set by government.

At an early stage, authorities need to establish a vision of where they are going and an explicit statement of the values or philosophy which guides their work. In addition, they should develop operational strategies for achieving long-term objectives. Another key function is to agree procedures for monitoring progress towards objectives and for keeping track of performance.

It follows from this that non-executive members will concentrate on policy-making and priority-setting and on working with the chairman and executive members to guide the purchasing and provision of services. The role and tasks of non-executive members will be different from those of former authority members. Nevertheless, certain statutory functions will still need to be undertaken.

Box 16   The Role of Authorities

Establishing overall policy direction and providing leadership

Developing a vision of where they are going

Agreeing operational strategies

Monitoring progress towards strategies

One approach is to delegate some of these statutory functions to committees and sub-committees to which authorities will be able to appoint lay people who are not members of the authority itself. The appointment of these people, who might be termed 'associates', will enable authorities to continue to fulfil defined responsibilities in relation to such functions as Mental Health Act duties in District Health Authorities and service committee hearings in Family Health Services Authorities.

Regional Health Authorities, District Health Authorities, Special Health Authorities, and Family Health Services Authorities will continue to be subject to the Public Bodies (Admission to Meetings) Act, 1960. This means that any formal meeting of the full authority must be open to the public, except where the authority resolves to exclude the public because of the confidential nature of the business to be discussed. Guidance from the Department of Health has made it clear that authorities will be expected to conduct their business in as open a manner as is reasonable.

In going about its business, each authority will have to decide how it wishes to work. This includes considering the balance to be struck between formal meetings (where authority decisions will be made or ratified) and informal meetings, the use to be made of committees and time-limited issue groups, and the information requirements of non-executive members. Authorities will also have to decide which matters to reserve for themselves and which issues should be delegated to managers or associate members.

There is no formal training for members, although the Department of Health usually runs seminars for new chairmen. In addition, the King's Fund College, the National Association of Health Authorities and Trusts (NAHAT), and other organizations offer a range of briefing and support activites. NHS authorities also provide briefing papers and seminars for new members.

Box 17 Briefing and Support for NHS Authorities

Seminars on specific issues for chairmen and executive and non-executive members

Policy briefings on major initiatives in the NHS

Support to individual authorities to clarify roles and relationships

Chairmen of authorities receive remuneration. From January 1991, Regional Health Authority chairmen will receive £19,110. Payments to district chairmen will vary from £13,812 to £17,610 and payments to Family Health Services Authority chairmen will vary from £9,903 to £11,510, depending on the size of authorities. Non-executives on Regional Health Authorities, District Health Authorities, and Family Health Services Authorities are paid £5,000. Both chairmen and non-executive members may also claim expenses incurred in carrying out their duties.

NHS Trusts

Many of the above comments apply to NHS Trusts as well as to NHS authorities but in a number of respects the position in Trusts will be different. Each Trust will be run by its own board of directors, independent of district and regional management. The board of directors will consist of a non-executive chairman, who will be appointed by the Secretary of State, and an equal number of executive and non-executive directors.

There will be a maximum of five non-executives. Two will be drawn from the local community and appointed by the relevant Regional Health Authority and the rest will be appointed by the Secretary of State. Where a Trust has a significant medical teaching commitment, one non-executive director will be drawn from the relevant university. All the non-executives will be chosen for the personal contribution they can make to the effective management of the Trust and not to represent any particular interest group.

The chairman and non-executive directors will receive remuneration and expenses for this work. In the case of chairmen, payments range from £13,812 to £17,610, depending on turnover. Non-executive directors will receive the standard fee of £5,000.

The executive directors will include the chief executive, the director of finance, and, for Trusts providing direct patient care, a medical and nursing director. The chairman and non-executive directors will appoint the chief executive, and they, together with the chief executive, will appoint the other executive directors.

All the directors will be full and equal members of the board and be responsible for determining the overall policies of the Trust, monitoring the execution of the agreed policies, and maintaining the financial viability of the Trust. The directors will not be personally liable for the actions of the board.

The Government has made it clear that it expects Trusts to be as open as possible in their management. As much of their business will relate to contractual and personnel issues they will not be required to open their routine meetings to the public or the Community Health Council. However, Trusts will be required to hold an annual meeting open to the public, at which a report on the previous year's performance and the audited annual accounts will be presented. Trusts will also have to hold a public meeting if an audit report is issued in the public interest at any time other than at the end of the financial year.

Trusts will, like health authorities, be able to delegate work to committees and sub-committees and to appoint lay people who are not on the board of directors to these

Quality Management

Following the Griffiths reforms of 1983, authorities have been expected to make quality a priority for all services provided to consumers. In part, this has been manifested in management strategies in which authorities have sought to make services more responsive to consumers. A variety of local initiatives have been taken in this area including surveys of patient satisfaction, the provision of information to patients about the services available, and an investment in staff training. Some authorities have also appointed senior managers to

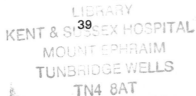

take responsibility for quality assurance and consumer relations. Particular emphasis has been placed on improvements to the environment of care and on ensuring that patients are treated as individuals.

More recently, *Working for Patients* emphasized the need to improve the quality of both clinical and personal care and this has led to action by the NHS Management Executive. Many authorities have developed their own quality initiatives and, in addition, central funds have been allocated for a programme of national demonstration projects focusing on three main areas.

Box 18 Central Quality Initiatives

Total quality management *

Out-patient services

Accident and emergency departments

* This is a management approach which aims to improve quality by putting the customer at the centre of all health care activity.

About 30 projects are currently being funded in these areas, the majority being total quality management projects. The Chief Executive has asked health authorities to put in place quality improvement programmes for all services, with specific action plans to contribute towards their implementation.

To assist this process earmarked funds (£7.5m in 1990/91) have been allocated to Regional Health Authorities and Special Health Authorities to support local projects in five target areas. These areas are:

☐ improvements to the physical environment and buildings
☐ schemes to assess the quality of services provided, including consumer surveys
☐ schemes to provide a more personal service
☐ improving information to patients
☐ staff training in quality issues.

The central importance of quality has been reinforced through the Management Executive's reviews of Regional Health Authorities' performance. Quality management has been a key issue addressed through the review process. In turn, Regional Health Authorities are expected to ensure that a quality assurance programme is being implemented in each District Health Authority and Family Health Services Authority within their area of responsibility. The system of management reviews and individual performance review (IPR) for managers are the main means by which objectives and targets for quality are set and their implementation monitored.

The Government's NHS reforms have also focused attention on how contracts between purchasers and providers can be used to raise standards. Guidance issued by the Department of Health identifies a number of aspects of quality that could be included in contracts.

Box 19   Aspects of Quality in Contracts

The appropriateness of treatment and care

Achievement of the optimum clinical outcome

All clinically recognized procedures to minimize complications and similar preventable events

An attitude which treats patients with dignity and as individuals

The environment conducive to patients' safety, reassurance, and contentment

Speed of response to patient needs and minimum inconvenience to them (and their relatives and close friends)

The involvement of patients in their own care

As the Government has acknowledged, it will take time to develop a range of quality measures for inclusion in contracts. To begin with, attention is likely to focus on conformity with legal requirements, national codes of practice, and standards developed by professional bodies and groups representing consumers. Examples of how authorities are dealing with quality in contracts are provided in the Department of Health's report, *Contracts for Health Services: Operating Contracts*.

In parallel, Family Health Services Authorities have a responsibility to improve quality in the family doctor service. Family Health Services Authorities discharge this responsibility by:

☐ visiting surgeries
☐ approving the hours of contact with patients
☐ allocating funds for the employment of practice staff and the improvement of doctors' premises
☐ ensuring that those providing specialist services (such as minor surgery) have the necessary experience, training, and facilities
☐ approving and monitoring the use of deputizing services
☐ providing information to the public
☐ carrying out consumer surveys and hearing patients' complaints.

A major aim of the NHS reforms is to strengthen the ability of Family Health Services Authorities to carry out these functions.

Family Health Services Authorities have more limited powers in respect of other family practitioners. The Dental Practice Board is responsible for clearing as appropriate all dental treatment before authorizing payment. Prior approval is required for certain complex and costly treatments. The Dental Reference Service undertakes quality checks, primarily in cases of concern. Dental practice advisers are currently being piloted in a number of Family Health Services Authorities as an additional means of improving the quality of dental treatment. The Royal Pharmaceutical Society of Great Britain undertakes quality checks of dispensed drugs on behalf of Family Health Services Authorities.

Doctors and nurses as well as authorities and their managers have taken an increasing interest in quality. A number of the Royal Colleges have undertaken special studies designed to improve performance. One example is the confidential enquiry into peri-operative deaths (CEPOD) undertaken by surgeons and anaesthetists. The confidential enquiry into peri-operative deaths showed that standards were generally high but a number of areas for improvement were identified. These included closer supervision of junior doctors by consultants, joint assessment of patients by surgeons and anaesthetists before surgery, and more systematic self-assessment by consultants.

Working for Patients makes clear the Government's aim to make medical audit part of the work of all doctors. In co-operation with the

Department of Health, all medical Royal Colleges have established or are in the process of establishing medical audit units. These units will develop standards and audit techniques that can be applied nationally. Health authorities and Family Health Services Authorities have received funds for the development of medical audit to help pay for staff costs, training, and investment in information technology.

Further Reading

Griffiths, R. (1983), *NHS Management Enquiry Report* (the Griffiths Report), DHSS, London.

Ham, C., Huntington, J. and Best, G. (1990), *Managing with Authority*, National Association of Health Authorities and Trusts, Birmingham.

Department of Health (1990), *Contracts for Health Services: Operating Contracts*, HMSO, London.

4 | Financing Health Services

The financing of health services is rarely out of the headlines. So how exactly is the budget for the NHS determined, and on what basis are allocations made to NHS authorities? Also, what steps have been taken to increase the efficiency with which resources are used?

Spending on Health Services

Expenditure on the NHS in the UK has increased from £444 million in 1949 to a planned £29 billion in 1990. Rising prices account for most of the increase in spending. Allowing for inflation, expenditure has increased more than fourfold during the lifetime of the NHS.

Expressed as a proportion of gross domestic product (GDP), spending on health services has increased from 3.9 per cent in 1949 to over 6 per cent in 1989. As Figure 6 shows, expenditure on health

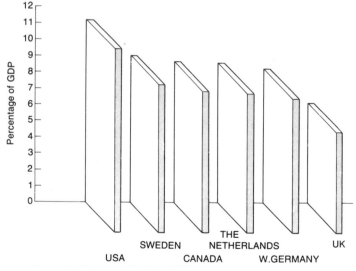

Source: Schieber and Poullier (1989)

Figure 6. Total Health Expenditure as Share of Gross Domestic Product, 1987.

44

services in the UK consumes a smaller proportion of gross domestic product than in many other developed countries.

The bulk of expenditure on health services in the UK derives from public sources. Although private expenditure has increased during the 1980s, it comprises a smaller proportion of total health expenditure than in most other countries.

Most of the money for the NHS derives from taxes followed by NHS contributions and income raised from charges and other receipts. The main charges are for prescriptions issued by GPs and dentists and for adult dental examinations and treatment.

The amount of money spent on the NHS each year is determined in the annual Public Expenditure Survey. This involves negotiations between the Department of Health and the Treasury. The outcome of these negotiations is announced in the Chancellor's Autumn Statement and full details are published in the Public Expenditure White Paper.

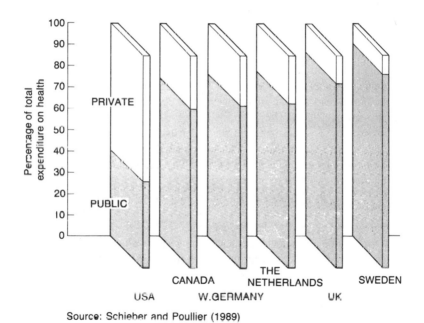

Source: Schieber and Poullier (1989)

Figure 7. Public and Private Expenditure on Health as Share of Total, 1987.

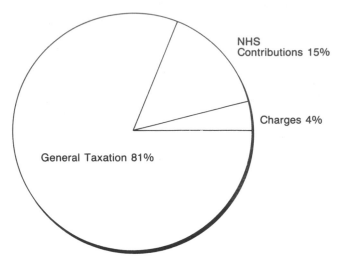

NHS
Contributions 15%

Charges 4%

General Taxation 81%

Figure 8. Sources of NHS Finance.

Currently, health services consume about 13.5 per cent of total public expenditure.

Table 1 sets out the plans contained in the 1990 White Paper for England. As the table shows, over 70 per cent of expenditure is on the hospital and community health services, 25 per cent is on the family health services, and the remainder is allocated to departmental administration and central health and miscellaneous services.

A more detailed breakdown of family health services expenditure is provided in Table 2. This shows that the biggest proportion of the family health services budget goes on pharmaceutical services, followed by payments to GPs, dentists, and opticians.

Health authority expenditure on different patient groups is illustrated in Figure 9. This shows the largest share of expenditure going on acute hospital services, and the smallest share going on services for children and mentally handicapped people.

Staff salaries and wages are the biggest single item of expenditure for the NHS as a whole, comprising 70 per cent of the total. Table 3 provides a breakdown of staff in different groups. As well as these directly employed staff, 25,300 GPs, 15,100 dentists, and 11,500 opticians are employed as independent contractors. There are also 10,100 retail pharmacists.

46

Table 1. Department of Health and Office of Population Censuses and Surveys – Cash Plans.

£ million

	1984–85 outturn	1985–86 outturn	1986–87 outturn	1987–88 outturn	1988–89 outturn	1989–90 estimated	1990–91 plans	1991–92 plans	1992–93 plans
Department of Health									
Central government's own expenditure									
National Health Service									
Voted in Estimates									
Hospital, community health and related services									
Current expenditure	9,122	9,607	10,325	11,402	12,640	13,659	14,810	15,540	16,190
Capital expenditure	767	803	820	807	817	920	1,085	1,110	1,110
Total	9,890	10,410	11,146	12,210	13,456	14,579	15,895	16,650	17,300
Family practitioner services									
Current expenditure	3,083	3,266	3,501	3,893	4,389	4,722	5,338	5,860	6,350
Capital expenditure	7	10	12	10	12	15	48	20	20
Total	3,090	3,275	3,513	3,903	4,401	4,738	5,386	5,880	6,370
Departmental administration									
Current expenditure	103	115	124	129	138	179	203	210	210
Capital expenditure	1	7	12	7	11	10	11	10	10
Total	104	122	136	136	149	189	214	220	220
Central health and miscellaneous services									
Current expenditure	285	317	348	379	380	420	448	470	490
Capital expenditure	18	22	22	14	19	22	22	20	20
Total	303	340	370	393	399	442	471	490	510
General Practice Finance Corporation									
Current expenditure					−8				
Capital expenditure					−8				
Total									
Total voted in Estimates	13,387	14,147	15,165	16,642	18,397	19,947	21,956	23,240	24,410

Table 1. *continued*

	1984–85 outturn	1985–86 outturn	1986–87 outturn	1987–88 outturn	1988–89 outturn	1989–90 estimated	1990–91 plans	1991–92 plans	1992–93 plans
Other (non-Voted)									
Hospital, community health and related services									
Current expenditure	−2		−5		−8				
Capital expenditure	−1		−8						
Total	−3		−13		−8				
Family practitioner services									
Current expenditure		−1		−4					
Departmental administration									
Current expenditure	13	14	14	14	15	15	15	20	20
Central health and miscellaneous services									
Current expenditure	−1	−1		−3	−1				
Capital expenditure				−1					
Total	−1	−1		−4	−1				
General Practice Finance Corporation									
Capital expenditure					−12				
Total					−12				
Total other (non-Voted)	9	12		7	−7	15	15	20	20
Total National Health Service									
Current expenditure	12,603	13,317	14,308	15,811	17,561	18,995	20,814	22,090	23,260
Capital expenditure	793	842	858	838	830	967	1,168	1,170	1,160
Total	**13,396**	**14,159**	**15,165**	**16,649**	**18,391**	**19,962**	**21,982**	**23,260**	**24,430**

Source: HM Treasury

Please note that figures are rounded and therefore may not sum to totals.

Table 2. Family Health Services Gross Current Expenditure, 1988/89 (England).

	Expenditure (£ million)	Expenditure as % of gross current expenditure on the family health services
General medical service	1,400	29
Pharmaceutical service	2,254	46
General dental service	950	19
General ophthalmic service	170	4
Family health services administration	103	2

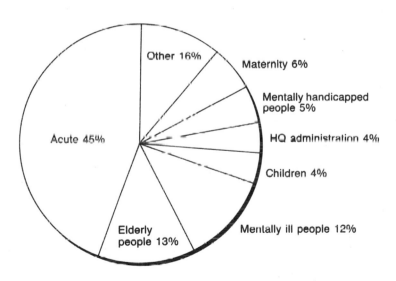

Figure 9. Health Authority Expenditure by Patient Group, 1988/89.

49

Table 3. Hospital and Community Health Services Staff, England.

thousands

Years	1978	1979	1980	1981	1982	1983	1984	1985	1986	1987	1988	1989
Medical and dental (including locums)	38	39	40	41	41	42	42	43	43	43	45	46
Nurses and midwives (including agency staff)	351	358	370	392	397	397	397	401	403	404	404	405
Professional and technical (excluding works staff)	57	60	62	65	67	69	73	74	76	79	80	80
Administrative and clerical	100	103	105	109	109	110	110	111	111	115	116	117
Works professional	6	6	6	6	6	6	6	6	6	6	6	6
Ambulance (including officers)	18	17	18	18	18	18	18	18	18	19	19	19
Maintenance	20	20	21	21	21	21	20	20	19	18	17	17
Ancillary	172	172	172	172	171	166	152	139	124	115	108	104
Total staff	**762**	**775**	**794**	**824**	**831**	**829**	**819**	**813**	**802**	**799**	**793**	**793**
of which: Direct care staff	446	458	472	498	506	508	512	518	522	526	528	530
Direct care staff as a percentage of total	58.6	59.0	59.5	60.4	60.9	61.3	62.5	63.8	65.1	65.9	66.6	66.9

Source: Department of Health

Please note that figures are rounded and therefore may not sum to totals.

Allocating Resources to Health Authorities

From 1992 – 93 Regional Health Authorities will be allocated resources by the Department of Health according to a formula based on the size, age, and health of their resident population. An allowance will also be made for the higher costs of providing services in the Thames Regions.

The aim is to achieve a smooth transition to the new system of funding, starting in 1990 – 91. As part of this, Regional Health Authorities will pay each other for those of their residents treated outside the region through adjustments in allocations made centrally. In 1991 – 92, District Health Authorities will contract directly with hospitals for these services and will pay hospitals through contracts. Table 4 illustrates the cash allocations to Regional Health Authorities in 1990/91.

Table 4. Regional Allocations (in £s million), 1990/91.

Regional Health Authority	Total revenue allocation	Capital allocation
Northern	911	51.4
Yorkshire	1024	61.0
Trent	1275	75.8
East Anglian	558	32.9
NW Thames	1058	50.7
NE Thames	1301	57.4
SE Thames	1164	59.3
SW Thames	933	48.9
Wessex	778	52.4
Oxford	614	36.9
S. Western	919	55.7
W. Midlands	1458	91.3
Mersey	723	39.1
N. Western	1238	73.5
Total	**13955**	**786.3**

Although most of the money allocated to health authorities takes the form of block grants, some resources are set aside by the Department of Health for spending on specific purposes. Notable examples in recent years include the waiting list initiative, the AIDS programme, services to combat drug misuse, funds for developing GP practice teams and improving premises, and joint finance money. The aim of earmarked allocations is to promote national policies identified as priorities by ministers.

Regional Health Authorities allocate resources to District Health Authorities. In the past District Health Authorities have been funded as providers of services in their units, but from April 1991 they will be funded to purchase services for their resident population. Initially, the resources received by District Health Authorities will reflect the cost of services currently being provided to each district's population. The way in which this is calculated for 1991/92 is summarized in Box 20.

Box 20 Allocating Resources to District Health Authorities

In 1991/92 allocations are based on:

a. A district's existing revenue allocation

b. *minus* the cost of providing services to the residents of other districts

c. *plus* the cost of services provided in other districts to the district's own residents

Funding District Health Authorities as purchasers rather than providers will result in significant changes in the resources received by some health authorities. In general, District Health Authorities are expected to use their allocations to support existing patterns of patient referrals except where they identify that changes are desirable and those changes can be planned and managed. This is the start of health authorities negotiating improvements in the way services are provided if they feel they can obtain a better service for their residents elsewhere.

In the longer term, the aim is to fund District Health Authorities on a weighted capitation basis. This will involve the use of a formula similar to that employed by the Department of Health in allocating resources to Regional Health Authorities. In other words, the funds received by districts will be based on the size of the population adjusted for age, morbidity, and any special local factors (e.g. deprivation).

Guidance issued by the Department of Health makes it clear that regions will have discretion in determining precisely how to allocate funds, subject to the following principles:

☐ there should be an emphasis on clarity, simplicity, and stability in the allocation mechanism

☐ the allocation mechanism should be the subject of consultation with districts in advance of its application, and made known and explicit

☐ funds should as far as possible go directly to districts in accordance with an agreed transitional pattern

☐ there should be clarity in the funding of districts as purchasers with a proper measure of financial responsibility at district level.

The Department of Health has also stated that Regional Health Authorities will retain the ability to earmark or topslice funds for specific purposes, for example to support training, but they will be expected to use topslicing selectively.

In practice, it is likely to be a number of years before District Health Authorities are fully funded on a weighted capitation basis. The new method of allocation will be phased in gradually to avoid further major changes in the money available to District Health Authorities.

District Health Authorities receive separate revenue and capital allocations. Capital expenditure controlled directly by District Health Authorities covers items such as minor building work. Bigger items such as new hospital schemes have to be paid for through capital allocations controlled by the Regional Health Authorities. Resources for major capital schemes are allocated in response to the plans published by District Health Authorities.

Income from land sales has been an increasingly important source of funds for capital developments in recent years. The rules on the use of this vary between regions but there is usually an arrangement in which a district receives some of the proceeds and the remainder is used for the benefit of the region as a whole.

Funding the Family Health Services Authorities

Family Health Services Authorities currently receive funds from the Department of Health to cover their management costs and to support improvements in practice premises and practice team staff. These funds are cash-limited. From April 1991, Regional Health Authorities will be responsible for allocating these funds to Family Health Services Authorities. In addition, Regional Health Authorities will work with Family Health Services Authorities to develop GP fund-holding, to determine budgets for GPs accepted as fund-holding practices, and to establish indicative prescribing allocations.

Family practitioners are paid by Family Health Services Authorities under the terms of nationally negotiated contracts. In the case of general practitioners (GPs), 60 per cent of income derives from capitation payments. The balance is made up of a variety of fees and allowances together with target payments for vaccination and immunization and cervical cytology smears. GPs also receive payments in respect of premises and practice team staff.

In the case of dentists, the new contract includes capitation payments for the care and treatment of children. Payments for adults with a continuing care arrangement are a combination of item of service and continuing care allowances. Other treatment is on an item of service basis.

Retail pharmacists are paid according to the number of NHS items dispensed. Pricing is the responsibility of the Prescription Pricing Authority which dealt with about 350 million prescriptions in England in 1988. Opticians receive a fee for NHS sight tests. Patients on low incomes receive a contribution towards the cost of their test and the making up of any spectacles they need.

It should be noted that the payments to family practitioners under the terms of their contracts are not cash-limited. Actual expenditure is determined by how practitioners decide to treat patients. This includes the prescribing of drugs, the carrying out of tests, the use of health promotion clinics, and the provision of dental care and treatment.

Efficiency Initiatives

Government policy in recent years has emphasized the need to increase the efficiency with which resources are used. A series of initiatives has been taken, including:

Cost improvement programmes

These are measures aimed at improving the use of resources by reducing the cost of running a service while achieving the same, or higher, levels of service output. The programme achieved annual savings in the hospital and community health services estimated to total £964 million between 1984 and 1990.

Income generation

This initiative was launched in 1988 to explore ways in which health authorities could generate additional income. £10 million was yielded in the first year through schemes such as income from private patients, car parking charges, and the use of hospital premises for retail developments.

Health service indicators

These indicators enable authorities to compare their performance with other authorities using routinely collected statistics. The indicators demonstrate wide variations between authorities in service provision and efficiency and provide a basis for management action in individual authorities.

In addition to the savings achieved through these specific initiatives, the Government has pointed to the increase in the number of patients treated as evidence of improved efficiency. Table 5 illustrates the main changes in hospital activity in the period 1978–88.

Steps have also been taken to increase efficiency in the family health services. Policy initiatives in this field include:

☐ the use of a limited list of drugs that GPs can prescribe
☐ the use of local formularies
☐ the introduction of indicative prescribing amounts for GPs
☐ the setting of financial incentives to encourage GPs to provide certain services.

Changes to the composition of Family Health Services Authorities and the appointment of general managers are also intended to ensure that the resources allocated to the family health services are deployed efficiently.

Table 5. Hospital Activity Statistics, England.

	1978	1979	1981	1983	1985	1986	1987–88	1988–89 (provisional)	thousands Annual average percentage change 1978 to 1988–89	1986 to 1988–89
Acute, geriatric and younger disabled										
In-patient cases treated	4,356	4,423	4,749	4,892	5,155	5,198	5,383	5,342	2.0	1.2
Average length of stay (days)	13.3	13.1	12.1	11.6	10.8	10.4	10.0	9.8	−2.9	−2.7
Out-patients (new attendances)	6,708	6,686	7,003	7,302	7,651	7,737	7,622	7,560	1.2	−1.0
Accident and emergencies										
(new attendances)	9,170	9,197	9,464	9,950	10,403	10,532	10,880	10,984	1.8	1.9
Maternity										
Obstetrics out-patients										
(new attendances)	678	709	695	681	698	696	652	611	−1.0	−5.6
In-patient cases treated	731	783	796	803	852	862	899	894	2.0	1.6
Mental illness										
Occupied bed days	28,534	27,908	26,793	25,312	23,647	22,448	21,540	20,990	−3.0	−2.9
Out-patients (new attendances)	187	180	188	192	201	202	207	192	0.3	−2.1
Mental handicap										
Occupied bed days	17,020	16,558	15,697	14,703	13,297	12,436	11,660	11,080	−4.1	−5.0
Out-patients (new attendances)	3.2	2.6	2.5	2.6	3.3	3.0	4.1	3.4	0.7	6.3
All specialities										
In-patient and day cases	5,932	5,992	6,474	6,832	7,317	7,464	7,500	7,580	2.4	0.7
Out-patient, accident and emergency (new) (excludes GP figures)	16,747	16,774	17,352	18,127	18,956	19,171	19,366	19,351	1.4	0.4
Day case admissions	562	592	714	813	963	1,050	881	998	5.8	−2.3
Ward attenders	n/a	n/a	n/a	n/a	n/a	n/a	774	853	n/a	n/a

Source: Department of Health

Further Reading

HM Treasury (1990), Chapter 13, *The Government's Expenditure Plans 1990 – 1991 to 1992 – 1993*, Department of Health and Office of Population Censuses and Surveys, Cm. 1013, HMSO, London.

House of Commons Social Services Committee (1989), *Public Expenditure on Health Matters*, HC418, HMSO, London.

Working Paper No. 2 (1989), *Funding and Contracts for Hospital Services*, HMSO, London.

Department of Health EL (90) MB/22, *District Allocations*.

Schieber G. and Poullier J. P. (1989), International Health Care Expenditure Trends: 1987, *Health Affairs*, 8: 3, 169–77.

5 | Policies and Priorities

The Royal Commission on the NHS, in its report published in 1979, noted that:

> the demand for health care is always likely to outstrip supply and the capacity of health services to absorb resources is almost unlimited. Choices have therefore to be made about the use of available funds and priorities have to be set.

Priority-setting occurs both within government and in NHS authorities. One of the features of the NHS is the existence of a wide variety of priorities in different fields. These include:

☐ the development of breast cancer screening and the strengthening of cervical cancer screening
☐ improvements to maternity and neonatal services
☐ the reduction of waiting-lists and waiting-times and the expansion of specific acute services
☐ the development of services for elderly people, people with mental illness, mental handicap or physical disabilities
☐ the development of primary health care services.

These priorities have been established over a period of years. Detailed guidance has been published in White Papers on particular services and in planning guidelines.

Health Service Priorities

The most comprehensive recent statement of national policy was published in 1988. This distinguished between *policy aims* and *service objectives*. Policy aims set the direction in which services should develop, and service objectives are the tasks all authorities are expected to carry out to a common timetable. The Department of Health has emphasized that wide variations in the circumstances of individual authorities mean that the pace of change in major services will not be the same throughout the NHS.

Planning guidelines issued in 1989 reinforced the aims and objectives set out in the 1988 circular. In particular, ministers

Box 21 National Guidance on Policies and Priorities

HC(88)43 Health Services Development. Resource Assumptions and Planning Guidelines
HC(89)24 Health Services Development. Resource Assumptions and Planning Guidelines
EL(90)154 NHS Priorities in 1991/92

announced that they wanted to see continued progress in improving the health of the population through:

☐ the prevention of illness and promotion of health
☐ ensuring the availability, in line with the structure for community care announced by the Government in its response to the Griffiths Report, of a range of services in settings which are best suited to the needs of patients and which reflect their wishes
☐ the effective diagnosis and treatment of illness and injury within times that are both clinically acceptable and reasonable
☐ attention to quality in the delivery of all services.

More specifically, authorities were required to introduce quantified targets to improve the health of their population, to bring about measurable improvements in community services so that people were not moved out of institutional care until appropriate services were in place to meet their needs, and to ensure that acute sector activity rates kept pace with demographic changes.

Guidance issued to authorities in 1990 confirmed that the policy aims published in 1988 and 1989 would continue to provide the framework for planning. Two specific areas of importance identified in the guidance were:

☐ the reduction of waiting-lists and waiting-times to ensure that, as a minimum, no patients wait more than two years for admission by 31 March 1992
☐ the review of maternity and neonatal services to include specific targets for improvement.

Authorities were also informed that the major task for NHS management in 1991/92 was to ensure that the range of reforms introduced through the NHS and Community Care Act and the three White Papers were implemented effectively and with maximum benefit to patients. This included achieving integration between primary and secondary care.

Regional Health Authorities and District Health Authorities are expected to plan their services in the light of national policies and priorities. The precise form which planning will take in future is currently under review by the NHS Management Executive and general managers. It is likely that Regional Health Authorities and District Health Authorities will be required to establish strategic frameworks for the development of services and to produce annual plans showing how they intend to achieve specific objectives. Family Health Services Authorities will plan their services in a similar way and Regional Health Authorities will be responsible for co-ordinating the activities of District Health Authorities and Family Health Services Authorities. The basis for NHS planning will increasingly be District Health Authorities' and Family Health Services Authorities' assessment of the need for health care of their population. NHS Trusts and directly managed units will be required to produce annual business plans looking ahead three years.

In producing plans for local service development, District Health Authorities must consult with organizations representing the public, such as Community Health Councils. The Department of Health has also emphasized the need for District Health Authorities to collaborate with other agencies and interests. These include Family Health Services Authorities, GPs, local authorities, and the private health care sector.

Public Health

The need for a concerted approach to public health issues on the part of health authorities was highlighted in the Acheson Report of 1988. In response to the report, the Government asked health authorities to appoint a director of public health. Among the tasks identified for the director were:

□ to produce an annual report on the health of the population
□ to provide epidemiological advice to the District Health Authority and Family Health Services Authority on the setting of priorities
□ to plan services and evaluate outcomes
□ to develop and assess policy on prevention, health promotion, and health education, and
□ to co-ordinate control of communicable disease.

The director of public health also acts as chief medical adviser to the authority.

The Government's NHS reforms reinforce the role of public health. This applies particularly to the responsibility of District Health Authorities as purchasers of care. Public health doctors will play a key part in assessing the population's need for health care and in advising on the purchase of services to meet this need.

Health Promotion

Since the mid-1970s, government policies have included a commitment to health promotion and disease prevention. Many of the initiatives that have been taken have focused on changes in individuals' life-styles as a means of improving health. People have been encouraged to give up smoking, drink less alcohol, eat a balanced diet, and take more exercise. There has also been a renewed emphasis on vaccination and immunization.

In parallel, priority has been given to screening programmes for cervical cancer and breast cancer and efforts have been made to combat drug misuse and the spread of AIDS. The AIDS programme has been supported by the establishment of substantial earmarked funds (£128 million in 1990/91). Each health authority is required to publish an annual report on action it is taking with regard to AIDS, and specific service objectives have been set for Regional Health Authorities and District Health Authorities.

The Health Education Authority has a national role in the field of health promotion. This includes working in co-operation with health authorities. The Authority is seeking to establish mechanisms for the joint planning of health promotion and disease prevention programmes with the NHS.

Much of the work of family doctors and staff employed in the community health services is concerned with health promotion. One of the main objectives of the primary care White Paper *Promoting Better Health* is to encourage GPs to give greater priority to work in this field. It is for this reason that the new contract for GPs contains financial incentives for GPs who achieve target levels of vaccination and immunization and cervical cancer screening. GPs will also receive special payments for holding health promotion clinics and carrying out health checks on new patients. The new contract for dentists has been designed with similar aims in mind.

Primary Care

Primary care is the first point of contact with the NHS for most patients. The primary health care team, comprising GPs, nurses, social workers, health visitors, and other personnel, play a key part in looking after patients and acting as gatekeepers to hospital services. Primary health care services are more fully developed in the UK and are provided to a higher standard than in most other countries.

There are, however, a number of weaknesses, including variable standards of care, overprescribing of drugs, and difficulties for patients in making a complaint when things go wrong. The Government's NHS reforms are designed in part to tackle these weaknesses. Family Health Services Authorities have been given a stronger role in the management of family health services and will be expected to take action to raise standards. At the same time, indicative prescribing amounts for GPs are intended to exert downward pressure on drugs expenditure. Simplified procedures to handle both formal and informal complaints, coupled with a longer submission time, may also help patients who are dissatisfied with the services provided by family practitioners.

The most significant innovation in primary care is the introduction of GP fund-holding practices. The fund-holding scheme and the new contract should encourage GPs to do more work themselves and to reduce the demand made on hospitals. Also, by making Family Health Services Authorities responsible to Regional Health Authorities, the Government has begun the process of ensuring that health strategies cover both hospital and primary care. This should be reinforced locally as District Health Authorities consult GPs and Family Health Services Authorities about the pattern and quality of care they wish to see.

Acute Hospital Services

Acute services account for almost half of all expenditure on hospital and community services. Policy in this area has developed in a piece-meal way and there has been no clear statement of overall priorities.

One major concern has been the reduction in waiting-lists and waiting-times. Earmarked funds have been set aside to tackle waiting-lists and £33 million was made available in 1990/91. Of this sum, £20 million was allocated to Regional Health Authorities and Special Health Authorities for the treatment of patients in specialities where there are long waiting-times. The remainder was used to fund the recommendations of a management team commissioned by the Department to investigate the 100 worst waiting-lists.

Another concern has been to achieve targets for particular operations. Priority here has been given to the expansion of coronary artery bypass grafts, hip replacements, and cataract operations. In parallel, the Government has supported the development of supra-regional services. These are services which, in order to be clinically effective and economically viable, need to be provided in a very small number of centres.

In 1990/91, £60 million was earmarked for supraregional services. The services designated for this support at present are illustrated in Box 22.

An important objective in relation to acute services has been to increase the efficiency with which resources are used. This involves using day-patient and out-patient treatment as alternatives to in-patient stays, and encouraging doctors to examine their practices more closely to see if savings can be made and applied elsewhere. Increasingly too, hospital doctors are taking a more active role in the management of services, most notably through resource management.

Box 22   Supraregional Services

Choriocarcinoma services

Craniofacial services

Endoprosthetic services for primary bone tumours

Heart transplantation

Liver transplantation

Specialized liver services

National Poisons Information Service

Neonatal and infant cardiac surgery

Psychiatric services for deaf people

Retinoblastoma services

Spinal injury services

Stereotactic radiosurgery

In tandem with medical audit, resource management should enable doctors and managers to ensure that resources are used effectively and efficiently.

Maternity and Child Care

Statistics indicate that there have been significant improvements in the health of mothers and babies during the 1980s.

Box 23   The Health of Mothers and Babies

Perinatal mortality has fallen from 15.5 per thousand still and live births in 1978 to 8.3 in 1989

Infant mortality has fallen from 13.2 per thousand live births in 1978 to 8.4 in 1989

Maternal mortality has fallen from 0.11 per thousand still and live births in 1978 to 0.06 in 1988

Source: Department of Health

It should be noted, however, that these figures, covering England and Wales, mask wide variations between different regions and districts. There are also significant differences between social groups, the children of people in professional and managerial occupations experiencing lower rates of mortality than those in manual occupations.

Policy on maternity services involves the provision of services in the community (e.g. midwives and health visitors) and in hospitals. The latter encompasses round the clock maternity cover and specialist expertise in obstetrics and paediatrics. Accessible antenatal care and screening facilities are seen as vital in detecting risk factors, coupled with the provision of counselling when an abnormal fetus is identified.

The Government has emphasized that the way in which services are provided should reflect the wishes of women whenever possible. Particular importance has been attached to the provision of care appropriate to the needs of women from ethnic minority groups. These and other issues were addressed in three reports prepared by the Maternity Services Advisory Committee between 1982 and 1985 (*see* Further Reading). The reports offer valuable guidance to NHS authorities on good practices in maternity care.

A report from the House of Commons Social Services Committee in 1988 led to a number of initiatives by the Government. These include:

☐ proposals to develop a confidential enquiry into still births and deaths in infancy
☐ the establishment of regional epidemiological surveys of still births and neonatal deaths
☐ the appointment of at least one paediatric pathologist in each region.

A National Audit Office report published in 1990 reinforced the need for authorities to tackle mortality rates significantly above average, to adopt good practices more systematically, and to review the efficiency of service provision. Subsequently, NHS authorities were advised that maternity services were one of two major priorities for 1991/92.

In the case of child health services, changes taking place in primary care following the White Paper *Promoting Better Health* are intended to involve GPs more fully in child health surveillance. This includes the monitoring of growth and development, offering advice and support, and providing immunization. GPs work closely with health visitors in this process. The National Association for the Welfare of Children in Hospital has produced a charter for children in hospital setting out the needs and rights of children who are acutely ill and their parents.

Elderly People

People aged 65 and over comprise a growing proportion of the population. Most elderly people live at home and many are in good health. However, advancing age tends to bring more ill health, and health services expenditure on elderly people is much higher than expenditure on people of working age. This is reflected in the capitation payments made to GPs and in the allocations received by District Health Authorities, both of which are weighted by age.

Box 24   Per Capita Expenditure in £s on Hospital and Community Health Services by Age Group, 1986–87 (England)

Total (all ages)	215
All births	1,185
0 – 4	195
5 – 15	95
16 – 64	110
65 – 74	415
75 – 84	927
85 +	1,452

Source: HM Treasury (1989) and Department of Health.

People who are 85 and over are particularly heavy users of health services and the number of people in this age group is expected to grow significantly in the next 20 years.

The main aim of policy, as set out in national guidelines, is to secure a balance of services which:

☐ facilitate and prolong independent living in the community outside institutions, particularly at home

☐ keep to a minimum the number and length of any necessary episodes of hospital care

☐ provide the most satisfactory achievable quality of life and autonomy for those who need continuing care in hospital or a residential or nursing home.

The Government has stressed that NHS authorities should work closely with other agencies to provide an integrated range of services. These services include support to enable elderly people to remain at home, acute geriatric care and assessment on a general hospital site, rehabilitation for return to the community wherever possible, and continuing care in small, homely units, close to family and friends. Continuing care provided directly by NHS authorities has been supplemented in recent years by private and voluntary residential care and nursing homes, much of which has been funded by social security payments.

People with Mental Illness

Policies in this area stem from the 1962 Hospital Plan and the White Paper *Better Services for the Mentally Ill*, published in 1975. A recent summary prepared in response to a report from the Social Services Committee updated earlier guidance (*see* Further Reading). This reiterated the need to build up services within the community and to phase out those hospitals too old, too large, or too remote to form part of the pattern of services needed in future.

Particular importance was attached to the development of a comprehensive psychiatric service in every district. The essential elements of such a service were identified as community care in the form of day hospitals, community psychiatric nursing, and support services available in the patient's home. In addition, a range of hospital services are needed, including in-patient services for long-stay patients, local accommodation for some elderly patients, general hospital facilities for assessment and short-term treatment, and a psychiatric department providing in-patient, out-patient, and day-patient services.

The Department of Health has emphasized that these health services need to be complemented by provision organized by local authorities, voluntary organizations, and the private sector. To encourage this, a new specific grant will be introduced in April 1991. The grant will enable local authorities to increase the range of social care services available to people with mental illness. Allocations will be made to local authorities when Regional Health Authorities are satisfied that social services and health authorities have agreed on the social care needed. £21 million will be made available in 1991/92.

Planning guidelines require each district to have a 'care programme' to enable co-ordinated care to be provided for people chronically disabled by mental illness living mainly in the community. The care programme is intended to ensure that there are:

☐ systematic arrangements for assessing the health and social care needs of patients who could be treated in the community

☐ effective systems for ensuring that agreed health and social care services are provided to patients who can be treated in the community.

Guidance issued by the Department of Health has emphasized the need for inter-professional collaboration in the development of care programmes and for patients and their carers to be involved in the agreement of programmes.

Although the number of people cared for in psychiatric hospitals has fallen in recent years, these hospitals continue to play an important part in the treatment of mental illness. One of the aims of national policy is to improve standards in large hospitals. The Health Advisory Service assists in this process by visiting hospitals and reporting the results to NHS authorities.

The law relating to mental illness changed in 1983 with the passage of the Mental Health Act. The provisions of the Act affect in particular those patients who are compulsorily detained, comprising about 10 per cent of all patients who are admitted to mental illness hospitals. The Act resulted in the establishment of the Mental Health Act Commission which has a general responsibility to protect the rights of detained patients and to keep under review the exercise of the compulsory powers and duties conferred by the Act.

An important category of patients are those needing treatment under secure conditions, including mentally abnormal offenders. These patients have traditionally been accommodated in either the prisons or the special hospitals run by the Special Hospitals Service Authority. In recent years secure units have been provided in each region for the treatment of some of these patients.

People with Mental Handicap

Current policy stems from the White Paper *Better Services for the Mentally Handicapped*, published in 1971. A recent summary prepared in response to a report from the Social Services Committee updated earlier guidance (*see* Further Reading). This reiterated the need to build up services in the community and to reduce dependence on larger hospitals. Specialized care is needed by people with severe handicaps but as far as possible services should be provided in small homely units based in local communities.

There has been a steady decline in the number of beds in mental handicap hospitals in the last 20 years. Currently, around 30,000 people live in these hospitals. The National Development Team assists health and local authorities in improving standards in mental handicap hospitals and in developing services in the community.

The Government has argued that the closure of hospitals is not a primary aim, although the part played by mental handicap hospitals in service provision is likely to decline further as care in the community is expanded. Increasingly, services are taking the form of packages of social care for people living independently or supported in group homes or residential communities. The aim is to encourage the provision of services to individuals based on a multidisciplinary assessment of needs and involving participation of the individuals concerned, their families, and other carers.

The NHS will have a continuing contribution to make to service provision through providing both general support and specialized services. As in the case of services for people with mental illness, District Health Authorities are expected to collaborate with statutory and other agencies to develop a comprehensive and integrated range of services for people with a mental handicap.

People with Physical Disabilities

Planning guidelines require health authorities to develop plans for people with physical and sensory disabilities in conjunction with other statutory agencies. These services have received low priority in the past and only recently has the Department of Health acted to correct this. Issues which authorities have been asked to consider in drawing up their plans are summarized in Box 25.

An immediate service objective is for authorities to develop plans for the absorption by 1991 of the artificial limb and wheelchair service currently provided by the Disablement Services Authority.

Box 25 Planning Guidelines for Services for People with Physical and Sensory Disabilities

Authorities should plan services for people with sensory disabilities, brain injury, multiple handicap; services for young people in transition to adulthood; provision of a district-wide incontinence service, with a continence adviser acting as a focal point; provision of disability equipment, including orthoses, prostheses, and communication aids and appropriate back-up services; provision of adequate therapy and other similar services; ensuring information on services is available in an appropriate form for use by disabled people; and the training of staff to be aware of the special needs of disabled people.

Community Care

Services for elderly people and people with mental illness, a mental handicap or physical disabilities will be affected by the changes to community care brought about by the White Paper *Caring for People* and the NHS and Community Care Act. These changes give local authorities the main responsibility in the development of community care, with District Health Authorities continuing to be responsible for hospital and community health services.

In future, local and health authorities will be required to draw up community care plans showing their strategic objectives, setting out their targets and priorities, and indicating how they will secure the services to meet the priorities identified in the plans. Local authorities and District Health Authorities, working closely with Family Health Services Authorities, must collaborate in reaching agreements on who will purchase which services for whom and at what cost. Some social care services will continue to be provided by local authorities but increasingly they will become enablers and purchasers, co-ordinating the provision of services in the public, private, and voluntary sectors.

One of the aims of the community care reforms is to achieve better value for the money spent in this area. In particular, there has been a huge increase in social security expenditure on private and voluntary residential care, providing an incentive to use this form of care instead of developing more appropriate domiciliary alternatives. By giving local authorities responsibility for assessing needs and transferring resources from the social security budget, the Government is seeking to enable more people to live at home for as long as they are able and wish to do so.

To work effectively, these arrangements require close collaboration between the staff who provide services and the agencies responsible for planning and purchasing services. The needs of those requiring community care span the responsibility of different agencies and only through a co-ordinated approach will it be possible to ensure that a seamless service is provided. This calls for strong leadership by NHS and local authorities and their top managers to promote an integrated strategy for service planning and service purchasing.

Ethnic Minority Health Care

The particular needs of people from minority ethnic groups have received increasing attention in recent years. A report produced by the National Association of Health Authorities and Trusts in 1988, *Action Not Words*, argued that NHS authorities should do more to meet the health care needs of black and other minority ethnic groups. This was reiterated in the Department of Health's planning guidelines issued in 1989. The guidelines asked authorities to take account of the needs of minority groups in preparing their plans and to ensure that these needs were met by a comprehensive range of services.

The new arrangements for contractual funding provide an opportunity for NHS authorities to look again at these issues. In particular, in assessing the population's need for health care, District Health Authorities and Family Health Services Authorities will be expected to examine the health problems of a multiracial and multicultural population. Also, the contracts that are negotiated with providers can be used to ensure that services are delivered in a way which is sensitive to the needs and concerns of black and minority ethnic people. This includes specifying within contracts a commitment to equal opportunities on the part of employers.

The Future

The rapid pace of change in health care technology will place increasing demands on health authorities in the future. Some examples will help to illustrate the possibilities.

The introduction of less invasive techniques will alter significantly the treatment of many conditions. These techniques have already had an impact, as in the use of flexible tubes such as endoscopes. Developments in fibre optics enable endoscopes to be passed into the body for investigation and treatment. Applications include the removal of gallstones and kidney stones.

A related development is the use of lasers. To date, lasers have been applied most effectively in eye surgery, the removal of skin blemishes, and by chest surgeons to clear airways blocked as a result of lung cancer. Other applications include treatment of lesions in the neck of the womb and as an alternative to hysterectomy in some cases. More experimentally, lasers have been used to clear blocked arteries.

An innovation which best illustrates the potential of the 'new surgery' is the lithotripter. This uses high-energy shockwaves to destroy kidney stones and it has revolutionized treatment in this field. Most patients with stones can be treated with a lithotripter and can be discharged within 24 hours of treatment. Research is now under way to evaluate lithotripsy for the removal of some types of gallstones.

Developments in the biological sciences will also have applications in the health services. As research progresses, it is anticipated that scientists will understand much more accurately the genetic contribution to diseases. This applies not only to specific inherited diseases like cystic fibrosis but also to some common illnesses such as heart disease, cancer, and strokes.

Related innovations hold out the prospect of producing specifically targeted anti-cancer drugs. This involves manufacturing monoclonal antibodies which attach to cancer cells. By coupling these antibodies to drugs which are effective in killing cells, the drugs can be accurately delivered where they are needed. Research into this kind of 'magic bullet' treatment is progressing rapidly, although practical success has so far been limited.

Major developments are also underway in radiology and pathology. In the case of radiology, these developments build on the introduction of computer assisted tomography scanners and magnetic resonance imaging. Using advanced techniques, doctors are able to build up sophisticated images of the body to assist both in diagnosis and treatment.

Similarly, a new range of tests in pathology will allow diagnosis for some conditions to occur at the patient's bedside, in the out-patient clinic, and in the GP's surgery. Also, an increased range of diagnostic kits may be available over the counter for self-testing. This is currently possible in the case of pregnancy and fertility tests, and other tests are likely to become available in future.

To ensure the proper use, application, and interpretation of results from these types of tests, careful control of usage and quality will be required. These developments could increase the demand for health services as individuals become more aware of the state of their health, and may require extra confirmatory tests to be performed by pathology laboratories.

Advances in health care technology may bring benefits to patients but they will add to the cost of health services. This is illustrated in Figure 10 which summarizes the resource implications of a number of medical technologies. In this situation, authorities will be faced with increasingly critical choices, and will have to weigh up carefully the costs and benefits of difference services.

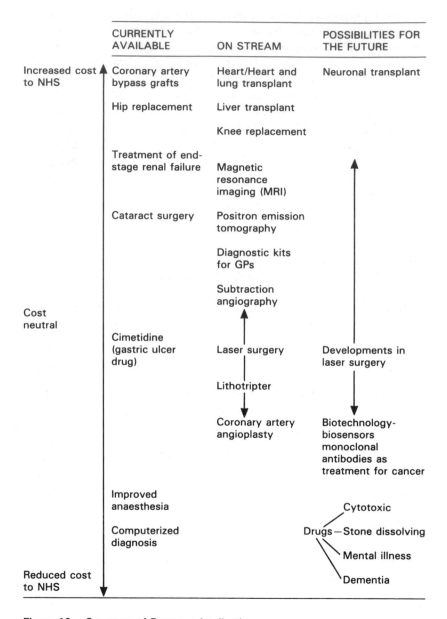

Figure 10. Summary of Resource Implications.

One approach to this is through the consideration of Quality Adjusted Life Years (QALYs). The Quality Adjusted Life Year is a technique which seeks to summarize in one measure the benefits of medical intervention in terms of the number of years of life they save and the quality of life saved. Information about costs can then be added and the cost per Quality Adjusted Life Year can be calculated. If this procedure is carried out for a range of treatments, it is possible to draw up a league table of the cost per Quality Adjusted Life Year of different treatments. When this is done, it can be shown that hospital dialysis is less cost-beneficial than renal transplants, while hip replacements or pacemaker implants are even better buys. It should be noted, though, that the use of Quality Adjusted Life Years remains controversial, and there is far from universal acceptance that they are a useful tool for determining priorities.

Box 26 Quality Adjusted Life Year League Table

Procedure	Present value of extra cost per QALY gained (£)
Pacemaker implantation for heart block	700
Hip replacement	750
Valve replacement for aortic stenosis	950
Coronary artery bypass grafts for severe angina with left main vessel disease	1040
Coronary artery bypass grafts for moderate angina with triple vessel disease	2400
Kidney transplantation (cadaver)	3000
Heart transplantation	5000
Home haemodialysis	11000
Coronary artery bypass grafts for mild angina with double vessel disease	12600
Hospital haemodialysis	14000

A number of health authorities have shown interest in Quality Adjusted Life Years as a tool for making expenditure decisions. However, it must be emphasized that Quality Adjusted Life Years are at an early stage of development, and a good deal of further work is needed to refine the method. There is also the ethical dilemma of placing a value on the life of others and denying treatment where it may bring benefit. In fact, this already occurs because it is not possible to offer treatment to all who need it with the resources currently available.

The proponents of Quality Adjusted Life Years argue that since rationing is inevitable it should be scientifically based in order to obtain the maximum benefit for the resources spent on health services. In this sense, Quality Adjusted Life Years are designed to help authorities make critical choices. While Quality Adjusted Life Years do not replace the need to make judgements, they do offer the potential of stimulating a more informed debate about priorities.

Analyses employing the Quality Adjusted Life Years methodology have tended to be confined to surgical operations and other procedures carried out in hospitals. The techniques of economic evaluation are nevertheless increasingly being applied to medicines. The Government's paper on the indicative prescribing scheme, *Improving Prescribing*, offered positive encouragement to pharmaceutical manufacturers to prepare cost-effectiveness and cost-benefit analyses to support their products. By examining outcomes as well as costs in this way, it should be possible to generate a more accurate assessment of the true resource implications of the use of any given medicine both for the NHS and the wider economy.

Conclusion

As the NHS approaches the end of the century, the challenges it faces are arguably greater than ever before. The ageing population, advances in health care technology, the move away from hospital into the community, and the emergence of new diseases such as AIDS will continue to tax the ingenuity and ability of those responsible for purchasing and providing health care services.

Achieving further improvements in health depends partly on the effective delivery of health services, but increasingly it calls for changes in personal behaviour and action by agencies outside the health field. NHS authorities have a major part to play in this process by:

☐ giving priority to health promotion, public health, and primary care services

☐ developing healthy alliances with local authorities and other agencies whose actions have a bearing on the population's health

☐ ensuring that within the health services priority is given to the efficient delivery of effective services.

It is easy to lose sight of these aims at a time when issues to do with the organization, management, and financing of health services dominate debate and discussion. However, unless NHS authorities are clear about the ends they are pursuing, expressed in terms of a vision for the future, then the opportunities created by the Government's reforms may be lost. Central to this vision should be objectives expressed in terms of the outcomes for the local population, involving either service improvements or health gains. Only in this way will it be possible to ensure that the real purpose of the reforms remains in view while authorities are grappling with the details of change.

Further Reading

HC(88)64, *Health of the Population: Responsibilities of Health Authorities.*

DHSS (1975), *Better Services for the Mentally Ill*, HMSO, London.

DHSS (1971), *Better Services for the Mentally Handicapped*, HMSO, London.

DHSS (1985), *Community Care: Government Response to the Second Report from the Social Services Committee, 1984–85 Session*, Cmnd. 9674.

Maternity Services Advisory Committee (1982), *Ante natal Care*, DHSS, London.

Maternity Services Advisory Committee (1984), *Care during Childbirth*, DHSS, London.

Maternity Services Advisory Committee (1985), *Care of the Mother and Baby*, DHSS, London.

Ham, C. *et al.* (1988), *New Horizons in Acute Care*, National Association of Health Authorities and Trusts, Birmingham.

Jennett, B. (1986), *High Technology Medicine*, Oxford University Press, Oxford.

Bosanquet, N. *et al.* (1989), *Will You Still Love Me?* National Association of Health Authorities and Trusts, Birmingham.

National Association of Health Authorities and Trusts (1988), *Action Not Words*, Birmingham.

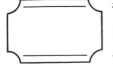

Useful Abbreviations

AIDS	Acquired Immune Deficiency Syndrome
CEPOD	Confidential Enquiry to Peri-operative Death
CHC	Community Health Council
CIPs	Cost Improvement Programmes
CMO	Chief Medical Officer
DGM	District General Manager
DHA	District Health Authority
DoH	Department of Health
DHSS	Department of Health and Social Security
DMU	Directly Managed Unit
DSS	Department of Social Security
FHSA	Family Health Services Authority
GDP	Gross Domestic Product
GP	General Practitioner
HAS	Health Advisory Service
HEA	Health Education Authority
IHSM	Institute of Health Services Management
IPR	Individual Performance Review
NAHAT	National Association of Health Authorities and Trusts
NHS	National Health Service
NAO	National Audit Office
NHST	National Health Service Trust
NHSTA	National Health Service Training Authority
PACT	Prescribing, Analysis and Cost Data
PEWP	Public Expenditure White Paper
PRP	Performance Related Pay
QALY	Quality Adjusted Life Year
RGM	Regional General Manager
RHA	Regional Health Authority
SHA	Special Health Authority
TQM	Total Quality Management
UKCC	United Kingdom Central Council for Nursing, Midwiffery and Health Visiting

Index

81